Elusive Fragments

Carolina Academic Press
Ethnographic Studies in Medical Anthropology Series

Pamela J. Stewart
and
Andrew Strathern
Series Editors

Elusive Fragments
Making Power, Propriety
& Health in Samoa

Douglass Drozdow-St. Christian

CAROLINA ACADEMIC PRESS
Durham, North Carolina

ISBN: 0-89089-746-8
LCCN: 2001096176

Carolina Academic Press
700 Kent Street
Durham, North Carolina 27701
Telephone (919) 489-7486
Fax (919) 493-5668
www.cap-press.com

Printed in the United States of America

Contents

List of Tables and Figures

Series Editors' Introduction

Pamela J. Stewart and Andrew Strathern

The overall aim of this series in medical anthropology is to provide a set of fresh texts which combine innovative approaches to general analysis with a strong grounding in classic ethnographic materials.

Medical anthropology is a vigorously developing sub-discipline within anthropology as a whole, and a related aim of the series is to produce works that show both the distinctive contributions of this sub-discipline and the ways it fits into the wider framework of the discipline at large.

The present work exemplifies these aims in a particularly apt and compelling way, the more so because of its emphasis on incidents from everyday life and what these reveal about wider cultural and historical themes. Samoan society has been the subject of many classic studies and of one long lasting controversy known as the Mead-Freeman debate, which revolve chiefly around questions of sexual practices. Drozdow-St.Christian resets the terms of this debate by fitting it into the more general framework of ideas about the body and embodied practice. He neatly gives his own solution to the contrary pictures drawn previously, by pointing out valid aspects of each side of the argument: Mead's picture reflected the ideas of some young, unmarried persons at a particular time, while Freeman presents the frameworks of discipline and social control that center on the morality of marriage and the family. Students of anthropology who read the present text will thus be given a new way of thinking about the issues set forth in the debate. In particular, the author's holistic approach will give his readers the opportunity to understand how a particular people think about and live with and through their bodies. Issues of bodily growth and health, maturation, sexuality and sexual identity, social rank and the use of space, punishment, bodily decoration, and finally illness and its treatment are all integrated together under this general framework.

It is here also that the author makes his personal contribution to the topic of medical anthropology. As an emergent sub-discipline of anthropology, medical anthropology covers many arenas and can be defined in various ways. We have explained and discussed a range of these definitions in the first book in this series, Curing and Healing: Medical Anthropology in Global Perspective (Strathern and Stewart 1999). While one obvious focus is on illness and its treatment, the correlative of this is clearly notions of health, and by taking as his theme the idea of the healthy body in its broadest sense, Drozdow-St.Christian gives us his own interpretation of what medical anthropology is about. There is room, of course, for many overlapping definitions and approaches here. Drozdow-St.Christian's own approach enables him to move across a spectrum of materials in an integrated way.

He also has his own theoretical approach through the idea of embodiment. This term has also come to mean various things in the usage of different authors. For some it has meant the inscription of social values on the bodies of persons. For others it has meant an emphasis on active and creative experience realized through the body. A chief exponent, in general terms, of this latter view has been Thomas Csordas, along with a number of others such as Michael Jackson and Paul Stoller. Drozdow-St.Christian in general follows this trend, while fusing into it his own vital concern with the affective sensibilities of bodily experience as a key constitutive element in social life. For him, embodiment is an important concept because it draws attention to how the Samoan person is grown and nurtured socially over time. By concentrating on this theme he also aims to discover how the body comes to be invested with meaning. He situates himself firmly here within a social constructionist view, noting how biological ideas of the body are themselves culturally informed, while at the same time reserving a space for personal creativity and experience in the development of meaning. In this way he also opens the way for a discussion of social changes, which he takes up explicitly in his Chapter 9.

For ethnography in general today historical change is another important point. Although Drozdow-St.Christian disavows an intention to write an historical account as such, stressing instead the contemporary scene itself, he is of course keenly aware that all phenomena are in a sense historically informed, including ideas about the body. His text provides ample illustration of this point, especially where he examines changing notions of sexuality, gender identity, body images, and illness in the context of the advent of AIDS as a disease, a point that applies throughout the Pacific and indeed globally.

Another significant theme for ethnography in general is the relationship between the particular and the general. The problems here apply at a number of different levels. Drozdow-St.Christian addresses the comment by Albert, his friend, who made a distinction for him between "facts" and "truth" — truth can be situational and facts are not meaningful unless set into their contexts. Generalizations are problematic and need always to be underpinned, and also modified, by situated observations. At a wider level, a similar point applies to the issue of making comparisons across cultural and social boundaries. Any study of Western Samoa is set against the backdrop of earlier studies, including those in American Samoa, and also the backdrop of the wider Pacific, including New Guinea. Drozdow-St.Christian's work contains some specific topics that are amenable to comparisons with specific areas of New Guinea, for example, although there are certain classificatory riskes in projecting these as comparisons with an overall category such as "Melanesia." Local diversities make such classifications difficult. This does not, however, preclude the work of comparison-making, as we have discussed in our study of "pathways of comparison" between Indonesia and Melanesia (Strathern and Stewart 2000). We can trace thematic threads of comparison across geographical areas and regions, finding correspondences but also differences that help to illuminate further individual cases as well as showing that these cases belong to more widespread patterns. Students reading this book may wish to think of its materials also in this light, so that Samoan trends and ideas can be compared with ones from elsewhere, and we give here some instances from New Guinea ethnography.

1) Christianity and Identity

"Christianity . . . is at the heart of contemporary Samoans' sense of their national and global identities" (Ch. 3).

Traditional religious beliefs and practices throughout the Pacific have incorporated Christian teachings (see J. Barker 1990 and Stewart and Strathern 2000), which have altered the ways in which the body is conceptualized in terms of its moral placement within religious doctrine and social practices.

In the Highlands of Papua New Guinea (PNG) Christianity has introduced new ways of evaluating self-worth as demonstrated through the decoration of the body. In the Hagen area of the Western Highlands Province women used to decorate their bodies with pig grease to make it shiny and to give it a healthy appearance. They also wore shell and marsupial fur decorative ornaments, displaying their affluence. Some of the churches taught that it was inappropriate to decorate the body in these ways and that the people should give the custom up to demonstrate adherence to the new religion. But nowadays decorating the body has taken on a renewed meaning as local dance groups exemplify regional forms of traditional body decoration and performing arts. Often these groups are sponsored by local churches as part of the formation of national identity in PNG today. Similar processes are at work throughout the Pacific region.

2) Genital Body Fluids

"Genital body fluids are not defined as either powerful or polluting by Samoans" (Ch. 4).

Much has been written in the Melanesian literature about genital fluids, which are seen as powerful substances that can be considered positively or negatively depending on whether they are thought to be in their culturally defined proper place or outside of it (see Stewart and Strathern 2001 for a discussion of bodily humors and substances in New Guinea). Menstrual blood is a fluid which is seen as a marker of a girl's maturity as a potentially reproductively active individual. This blood is thus a positive and poignant indicator of fertility. But menstrual blood is also thought by some New Guineans to be dangerous in other contexts. For example, in Pangia in the Southern Highlands of PNG men were afraid that if they took menstrual blood into themselves, either through their penises or inadvertently through ingestion, they could become impregnated and without a proper organ to give birth that they would become swollen and die. Special rituals were performed to heal a man who became sick in this way (Strathern and Stewart 2000). Such ideas indicate the importance for the people of the proper placement, as well as the proper flow, of powerful substances such as semen and blood. Drozdow-St.Christian has raised an interesting comparative point in this context.

3) Conception

"An open space around this organ . . . is the location for the combination of semen and the blood of the mother which results in the development of the foetus" (Ch. 4).

In the Hagen area (Western Highlands Province of PNG) conception is also seen as the mixing of semen and blood in an action in which the female blood is surrounded by the male's sexual fluid, a process that eventuates in the growth of a fetus if it is properly nourished in the womb by the mother (see Strathern and Stewart 1998 for a detailed description). The positive role of semen in producing a fetus is counterbalanced by semen's ability to "pollute" or "spoil" breast milk. Hence the taboo on sexual intercourse during postpartum breast-feeding years.

Ideas of how conception occurs are particularly interesting to think about nowadays in consideration of new forms of reproductive mechanisms such as those introduced through reproductive technologies in which many of the normative practices of sexual reproduction are transformed through medical interventions. These may not yet have entered into the lives of many Pacific islanders. If and when they do so, we can expect them to impact ideas about kinship in general. For many Pacific societies, nurturance is as important in defining kinship as are notions of genealogical connections, indeed such connections are themselves partly seen as aspects of nurturance or feeding. The impact of new forms of reproductive technology will therefore itself be modified by ideas of this kind.

4) Embarrassment and Self-Worth

"Making the penis visible, even in conversation, is, for many Samoan men, more fraught with embarrassment than discussing what it is the penis is used for" (Ch. 4).

The body, including the mind, is the seat of self-worth and the emotional expression of selfhood as expressed in relation to others. An example from the Duna people of the Southern Highlands Province of PNG demonstrates this point nicely. When two Duna men described how the neighboring Oksapmin men used to come on trading expeditions, bringing stone axes and other goods, it was said that they wore penis gourds. This was described to us with great laughter and embarrassment when it was explained that the men had their pubic hair and testicles exposed, a practice that the Duna did not adhere to. We were told that it was not appropriate to laugh at these men when they came but to divert oneís gaze was acceptable. Laughing at the men was said to bring illness upon the man who did so. Embarrassment and laughter were thus linked together but constrained by fear of the resentment of these Oksapmin "others" who were also linked to the Duna people as trading partners.

5) The Skin

"Skin, for Samoans is the ultimate and most intimate point of connection with the world, and at its most crucial, it is the only reliable 'text' for other Samoans to read the nature and quality of some other person. Skin is the public organ . . ." (Ch. 8).

The skin of the body can be seen as a map to the inner state of the person. For Hageners (Western Highlands Province, PNG) "shame" is said to be expressed and read on the skin. The skin mediates the outside and inside realms of the person, joining them together. It therefore becomes a sign that can be read both ways: as an indicator of inner states and of the social circumstances that underlie these inner states. Interestingly, Samoans like Hageners say that one cannot directly perceive or understand inner states themselves. But the body, and in particular the skin, becomes the means whereby the inner state of a person is made known to others.

6) Anger and Illness

Drozdow-St.Christian tells us that for Samoans, "Anger is both a cause and effect of illness, depending on the circumstances and the type of illness" (Ch. 8).

Like shame, anger can also be read on the skin through the sickness that it produces. Drozdow-St.Christian's account here makes it clear that the parallel with Hagen ideas noted above with regard to the skin applies with regard to anger also. In Hagen, a person's anger can cause illness to the person himself or herself. The sick person should then "confess" the anger and indicate its cause. Restorative attempts to remove the cause by payments of compensation and by sacrifices are then set in hand, and the sick person is then expected to recover (see Strathern and Stewart 1999 for a detailed discussion of this topic). Similar patterns appear to be working in the Samoan context, as when a sick man was given an expensive present of rugby boots by a relative who was said to have spoken badly of him. Nowadays, as in Hagen, Samoans also say that God may be angry with people and punish them with sickness. Clearly this is a different process from that given above, but it may not be new, since God may be here taking the place of the ancestors.

7) HIV and AIDS

"Many men spoke of how they felt like their power was being undermined by HIV/AIDS because it meant that they could no longer father strong children" (Ch. 9).

Sentiments of this kind demonstrate the strong connection which, as Drozdow-St.Christian points out, Samoans make between sexuality and reproduction in a gendered familial context. Again, such a reaction must be common throughout the Pacific and elsewhere. In Hagen, senior persons similarly deplore the possibility that younger people may simply die out because of AIDS and that the reproductive continuity of their society will be broken. Such an apprehension falls on people well before epidemic levels of the disease are confirmed and itself conditions their ability to think about the future. This is a fear equally shared between the genders.

We have given here just a few examples of how this book can be set into a wider regional context of comparisons. Drozdow-St.Christian's own main purposes are cogently explained throughout his text and especially at its beginning and end. The beginning stresses his wish to enliven ethnography through remaining faithful to bodily experience (while he recognizes that this too can be culturally variable). His last chapter gives a programmatic picture of how embodiment theory can improve our anthropological understanding of the world in general, including therefore questions of health and sickness. Along the way he often neatly sums up his ideas with remarks such as "Lived experience and culture are not distinguishable" (Ch. 2), or his plan to give an account of "fa'a Samoa ['the Samoan way'] from the body up" (Ch. 3); or his view that for the

Samoans there is no separate realm of the psyche since "everything is body" (Ch. 8). The body, as he presents it, is certainly good to think with and about, and the body of his text gives us much food for thought about what health and illness mean.

References

Barker, John (ed.) 1990. *Christianity in Oceania*. ASAO Monograph no. 12. Lanham, MD: University Press of America (Rowman and Little-field).

Stewart, Pamela J. and Andrew Strathern (eds.) 2000. *Millennial Countdown in New Guinea*. Special Issue of *Ethnohistory* 47:1.

Stewart, Pamela J. and Andrew Strathern 2001. *Humors and Substances: Ideas of the Body in New Guinea*. Westport, CT and London: Bergin and Garvey.

Strathern, Andrew and Pamela J. Stewart 1998. Melpa and Nuer ideas of life and death: the rebirth of a comparison. In M. Lambek and A. Strathern (eds.) *Bodies and Persons: Comparative Perspectives from Africa and Melanesia*, pp. 232-251. Cambridge: Cambridge University Press.

Strathern, Andrew and Pamela J. Stewart 1999. *Curing and Healing: Medical Anthropology in Global Perspective*. Durham, NC: Carolina Academic Press.

Strathern, Andrew and Pamela J. Stewart 2000. *The Python's Back: Pathways of Comparison between Indonesia and Melanesia*. Westport, CT and London: Bergin and Garvey.

7th September 2000
Whatriggs Farm, Newmilns,
Ayrshire, Scotland

Author's Preface and Acknowledgements: On Being a Body Out of Place

The past and present wilt—I have fill'd them, emptied them.
And proceed to fill my next fold of the future.

Listener up there! what have you to confide to me?
Look in my face while I snuff the sidle of evening,
(Talk honestly, no one else hears you, and I stay only a
minute longer.)

Walt Whitman: Song of Myself

My objective in writing this book is a simple one. I want to explore how power, propriety, and health, each of which are fundamentally social processes, are indivisible facets of the process of embodiment, that intensely cultural, cognitive, and phenomenological process of having a meaningful body and deploying it, in appropriate and meaningful ways in the world. Put another way, my purpose here is to give the culture of power and propriety and health in Samoa some flesh by demonstrating how embodiment is the fundamental social process which not only mediates the lived effect of culture but makes culture possible. But in doing so, there is the risk that issues of health in Samoa, issues of real morbidity and mortality may get abstracted to the wayside. In writing about health as cultural process, it is important we not lose sight of the political economies of who gets sick and who gets well, who dies and who does not. As Farmer [1999] argues eloquently, the most profound modern plague is the plague of inequalities. The argument I will advance here seeks to contribute to our understanding of this more pervasive plague by grounding health in the embodied relations and embodied social processes in which Samoans find themselves. By locating healthy bodies in a grounded ethnographic account of Samoan embodiment, with all that goodness, propriety, and health entail as social practices, the argument I advance here serves as a step both backwards and forwards, towards a comprehensive social and political economy of illness in Samoa and elsewhere.

xvii

My argument here is historically informed, though I am not attempting a reconstruction of Samoan bodies of the past. Where historical transformations can be readily excavated from living experience, I will explore how certain aspects of embodiment have changed in recent history. However, I am not advancing an historical argument here. Rather, I am interested in the processes, practices, and entailments of embodiment as they are being enacted in the Samoan social field today. That field is a confluence of historical processes and an approach which sought to locate a historical Samoan embodiment as well as a modern one would fall prey to a fundamental problem of substituting bodies fixed in time for the more fluid, transient and transcendent body that I refer to in referring to embodiment as a cultured and enculturing process. Time is never far from the surface of my discussion here, but changes through time are not the object of my enquiry. It is important, however, to not view the argument here as being an argument about historical changes. I hope to show there are enough changes and transformations in the processes of embodiment as a living thing, that seeking to unravel in any detail the longer history of these changes would cause this current book to spiral ever and ever larger.

Medical anthropology, while focussing on the cultural and socio-structural facets of disease, begins from the diseases themselves and works backwards to the socio-cultural, adopting many different perspectives which are outlined in more detail in *Curing and Healing: Medical Anthropology in Global Perspective* by Andrew Strathern and Pamela Stewart, the first volume of this series [Strathern and Stewart 1999]. What I am proposing here is a different orientation, one which starts from culture and in particular the processes and praxis of embodiment and works outward to disease. What I refer to here as health-making, that life long process of enacting a good and proper embodied presence, needs to be approached in its own right, in order to show how particular disease events are part of this larger process of being a healthy body in the world, rather than discrete things in themselves. What I am suggesting here is that Sontag's notion of the kingdom of the sick distorts the cartography of embodied presence by making of disease a process or event discrete from some other normal form of embodiment. I hope to show here that disease is part of an ongoing practice in which and through which appropriate posture, rules about urinating, and so on connect with models of disease and cure in a single poly-faceted making of healthy presence. In other words, while anthropologists have long concerned themselves with an analytic holism, I hope to show that this holism is not simply a theoretical or philosophical orientation or posture, but an integral aspect of social being, encultured and enculturing presence, and the multiple lives of history and society. Stepping back from healthy and diseased dichotomies is, for me, the first step in this re-orientation.

To accomplish this, I have laid out the book such that it arrives at illness and health making as part of a larger analysis of what goes into making, having, doing and being a good and proper body in Samoa. Section 1, *Landscapes,* explores this ground in two ways, looking in Chapter 2 at some theoretical and methodological issues which inform my discussions, and in Chapter 3, at an overview of Samoan society, culture and everyday life. These chapters are meant to orient the reader to issues I am addressing here, and to the character and quality of Samoa today. Section 2, *Inventions and Intentions,* explores the beginning phases of embodying praxis by looking at pregnancy, infancy and childhood. In particular, I focus on such things as Samoan 'toilet' training, the socialization of children into a socio-centric orientation to community life, and the moral and practical geography of eating and meals. In the next section, *Deployments and Constraints*, I examine various sites of social control, power, discipline, and the many transgressions that occur in and around the embodying practices of punishment and pleasure. From sex to spirit possession, these chapters describe the processes and practices through which the body is implemented and is an implement in the prosecution of both excess and restraint. The final section, *Peril, Preservation, and Change* looks closely at the way Samoans deal with what for them are the most dangerous and endangered of bodies, the sick body and its ramifying implications for the community as a whole. Illness in Samoa is not simply about doctors and patients, as Chapter 8 explains, and transitions in health and healthy bodies in Samoa reflect wide ranging implications for social change across the entire scope of *Fa'a Samoa* — the Samoan way, issues explored in Chapter 9. The final chapter, Chapter 10, returns to the theoretical and methodological issues raised in Chapter 2, this time relating them more closely to the ethnographic ground of Samoan embodiment, as a way of continuing the dialogue on our understanding of culture and society as both products and producers of meaningful and meaning generating bodies.

All ethnography is about developing composites, from field research, from the work of others in the places we are studying and elsewhere, and in the minutiae of analysis, reflection and interpretation which we engage in as anthropologists. In offering here what I like to think of as evocative composite sketches I want to connect the many and often varying accounts among informants in ways which do no violence to this variation while at the same time not ending up sounding like a Babel of particularization. And so each "fact" or "idea" is connected with and weighed up against other versions, other accounts, so that what finally emerges is something which is reasonable but not generic. In connecting varying accounts, the goal is to triangulate these accounts upwards from the details of each variation, to the core conceptual components around which these variations circulate.

Indeed, one way of thinking about composites is to think of the body as an accomplishment, that thing which you are currently using to hold, read, and think about these pages. At the same time, it is a densely complex network of processes which vary in detail between each of us. And so we can say, in a reasonably general way, that you are reading this text because light, reflected off the variations in colour on the page, are striking the wall at the back of your eyes and triggering electro-magnetic impulses along the optic nerve to specific centres in the your brain, centres which convert those impulses into mental images or sensations. That general observation does not negate the variation in eyesight, lighting conditions, the condition and efficiency of the optic nerve, or the way these interpretive centres in the brain convert the impulses into thinkable things. And it most certainly does not diminish the importance and effect of the histories, interests, and knowledges each of you bring to the processes of reading this text. Good ethnography seeks to convey all three, in their consistency and complexity, because culture, social life, history are always all of these things, and more.

For me, a musical model helps keep me focussed on the processes of fixity, balance, and permutation which ground ethnography. Bach's preludes and fugues revolve around a balancing between fixed codes and fluid performance. Bach's fugues are held together by the arrangement of harmonics which are vertical, chordal structures around which the variations of the fugue are arrayed in increasing or decreasing complexity. In some performances, for example those of the later Sviatislav Richter, these vertical harmonics are highlighted and given prominence, with the variations appearing to flow out from them as if the vertical lines were like military commands. In contrast, a recent performance by the young Russian-American pianist Sergey Schepkin pushes these harmonic sign posts into the background, letting the variations work almost by insinuation so that we hear the vertical harmonics without their being stressed. Each performance works, and in each the whole is held together by these vertical lines. One, however, stresses the variations, while the other stresses the order. *Fa'a Samoa* — The Samoan Way — is like a fugue in the sense that there are central codes and concerns around which variations and deployments are performed. The analysis of this system of fixed codes and expanding and contracting variation is like a performance of Bach's fugues in that it is possible to emphasize or insinuate the codes in their relationship to the variations. Equally, the living performance of *fa'a Samoa* can take either of these approaches, and often does. Stability and variation, order and exploration, norms and nuance — these are the qualities of *fa'a Samoa* I want to navigate within, in my own performance not simply of my understanding of Samoan praxis, but also in a performance of it — this text — that balances hard and fast with flexible and cursive.

So this is a composite, as rigorous as I can make it given the state of my understandings of Samoan life and culture. Rigorous, but always "not quite real." It is a speculation on the connections and disconnections, the continuities and otherwise-between core values and ideas, and the bodies on which, and through or because of which, they are engaged. Like a map, which is not after all made up of mountains and rivers but representations of them, what follows here is a representation, a rigorous figure of speech if you will, informed by my own concerns and interests which must not, in the end, be mistaken for those of Samoans themselves. I can only hope they will forgive me "sounding my barbaric yawp" over the roof of the world they live and understand so much more fully than I can hope for. But don't for a moment think I am saying this in order to distance myself from what follows, to somehow apologize for it. I am not. This is an anthropology of Samoa, it is not Samoa itself. I make no apologies for that, though I will first and always apologize to my Samoan family and friends for anything I have gotten wrong.

Where writing is a lonely art, thinking about Samoa has been an ongoing and communal process in which the influence and effort of so many people are deeply embedded, and embodied. My family and friends in Samoa were tireless in their pains to help me see and, they hoped often against all hope, understand what was going on around me. Their modesty forbids my naming them, other than to recall the welcoming embrace my late Samoan mother, Pai, gave me the first night I spent in Samoa, an embrace which continues to wrap me in memories of our endless hours shopping for the best sausages in Apia, or sitting on the sea wall outside the Tusitala hotel listening to the bands playing in the open aired bar inside. Many friends guided me, chided me, chastised me, and as my dearest friend Albert put it one day, showed me where to put my hands. Tia'i, with whom I spent some part of almost every day during my first year in Samoa, remain a presence watching me as I type these words. Julia and Sonny invited me to live with their family, when we first met in Canada. That is a kindness beyond gratitude, and I remain humbled by it. Mapesone, who became my most intimate friend on so many levels, and whose death recently I continue to feel like a jolt of vicious electricity through my heart, taught me how to be a whole new person, no small task for such a small young man. Rest well.

Where writing is lonely, publishing is always something done in teams. I have been lucky to work with the editors and technical consultants at Carolina Academic Press, and want to thank in particular Glenn Perkins and Leah Rutchick who, as my editors, managed to find the sense in my all to often mangled prose. I also want to thank the series editors, Andrew Strathern and Pamela Stewart, for their encouragement and for a couple of quite compelling reminders not only about who I am writing for, but also who I am writing about.

In Canada I have been guided, chided, and chastised by the best. Bill Rodman, who became my mentor and friend long before I ventured to Samoa, remains my mentor, friend, and now colleague. We've witnessed, taken part in, and survived so many of each others ups and downs. And I warn you, Bill, there is more where that came from. I won't even begin to name other colleagues, for fear of missing someone important, especially since they know who they are and they know—because I never tire of telling them—how important they are to me. But I must, and must always, recognize again the effect knowing Trish Wilson has had on my mind and on my soul. Her death left a crack in the face of the world, from which her light continues to warm me whenever I need to be warmed.

I have so many families. My mother, Mary, has encouraged me, been confused by what it is I do for a living, and then encouraged me again. My other family—Marlene, Nana, and Michael and Natasha and Trixie—have shared so much with me during this last decade and their affection is a source of nourishment and astonishment for me. Most importantly, they have shared their son, Stephen, who for 11 years, has been, and remains, the core of my own being in the world. Preposterous as we often are, dear boy, we are preposterous together.

Most of what I understand about being a body in Samoa comes from nearly a decade of personal reflection and experience, as part of the process of being incorporated into the Samoan families and communities in which I have studied. It is this, being a body out of place in someone else's social field, which is at the heart of my interest in understanding the living history of constructed bodies, not only in Samoa. Being a body out of place, recognizing and using that position as part of my analysis here, means that much of what is in this book is not only anthropology but something more intimate, more personal. I have engaged my own experiences of my own body being made into sense and sensibility not only by my self, but by the people around me, in order to strive for an incorporated understanding of "what it is like" to be hungry or tired or aroused or angry or sad or in pain, as a Samoan, in the world which Samoan bodies make for themselves. Ethnography, as I will argue over and over again in this book, has too often been a fleshless, bloodless, indeed lifeless thing. Where, in the pages that follow, I ascend to steeply into abstraction, it is always, I hope, with my feet still padding noisily along the muddy roads of Vaimoso, or my with my heart pumping loudly while chasing down a pig for a cousins wedding. What I want, more than anything else is to convey here is what someone else once called "the Samoan dance of life"—a dance that is stately, incongruous, brutal, passionate, funny, and deeply affectionate and vigorous. While I will always remain, in my experiences in Samoa, a body that does not quite fit, my faltering attempts at participating in that dance are done in respect and, most importantly, out of love for the people around me.

In all of this, I remain responsible—for omissions, errors, misguided interpretations, wrong headed good intentions and occasional lapses into bloody-minded stubborness. I am reminded of the next lines in the poem by Whitman with which I began this short preface:

Do I contradict myself?

Very well then I contradict myself,

(I am large, I contain multitudes.)

This can be said, with equal merit, not only about what I have written here, but about the large, ambiguous and lively world this book sets out to explore.

A Note on Pronunciation and Orthography

Samoan is a complex language, both when spoken and when written. A simple pronunciation key will help the reader with some of the Samoan words:

G [Gasegase]	pronounced	"ng" [singing]
ā,ē,ī,ō,ū	pronounced	long vowel as in father where week lone moon
a,e,i,o,u	pronounced	short vowel as in cut set sit bond put
' [glottal stop]	pronounced	as a slight tap before the vowel it precedes

Long and short vowels, as well as the glottal stop, alter the meaning of words.

eg: *tau*—deck of a fishing canoe and *tāu*—connected by kinship
ava—break in the reef and *'ava*—beard

As well, 'n' between two vowels is often pronounced 'ng' as in lagona [to hear or perceive] and lagoga [to weave a fine mat]. While this does not effect written Samoan, in speech such inconsistent variation allows for considerable punning and other plays on words. Vowel initial words with no glottal stop sound, to English speaking ears, as if they are being initiated with an 'h' sound, but this is a trick of the ear. As well, an 'i' following a short vowel adds the 'y' sound as in yes between the vowels [aiga = ai-yinga], while a short vowel following a 'u' is seperated by a 'w' sound [aua = ow-wa], although these are not actually present in the spelling of the word. All vowels are pronounced in Samoan words, though contiguous vowels are often blurred into what appears to non-Samoan speakers to be a single sound [tau = taoo but sounds like tou as in out]. Unlike glides in English, however, both vowels are distinctly, though quickly, pronounced.

Elusive Fragments

Chapter 1

A Prologue: Nights and Days in the Kingdoms of the Sick

Se'i lua'i lou le 'ulu taumamao
(First, pick the highest breadfruit)

Samoan Proverb

I woke through the night, less than a week after arriving in Western Samoa, wet from cold sweat. So wet in fact that the slight breeze from the louvred windows had set me shivering, the shivering waking me with a start. Somewhere in the night a rooster crowed very slowly. My house was surrounded by a darkness made complete by the clouds which covered the moon, and through the windows I could make out only vague unidentifiable shapes, of the trees moving in the breeze, of the houses nearby, of a cache of lava rocks which marked the bank of the Gasegase Stream. Somewhere someone coughed, lost in the darkness so that the sound seemed to come from everywhere at once. I turned slowly away from the window, pulling the damp sheet with me and began to curl into a compacted ball, a wrenching cramp in my groin twisting my legs until they were almost under my chin. The shivering stopped and I lay so still the tremor of my breathing made the bed vibrate.

Earlier that day, as I was a newcomer to the village and ignorant of the beauties and wonders of Samoa, members of what would become my adoptive family had taken me on a driving tour across the main island of Upolu to Togitogiga National Park. The park rises slowly up from the western coast of Upolu through a narrow volcanic valley through which a chilled stream runs. It is a favourite spot for family picnics, especially on religious holidays. Manicured miniature Samoan *fale* [thatched roof, open walled traditional houses] sit among tailored trees overlooking the narrow gorge through which the stream enters the sea. Several women, charged that day with cleaning up rubbish after a heavy rain storm, sat in one of the *fale* drinking tea from a metal kettle and talking. It was the first time since my arrival earlier in the week that I had heard people talking together in Samoan, the family I was living with adopting English [in which all but the youngest son was fluent] to, they told me, help me feel like I was home. The simulated Samoan houses, the softly laughing women in bright *lavalava*, the murmur

3

of the stream as it splashed slowly through the gorge. Some god of welcome, or perhaps of irony, had created a post-card miniature of South Pacific stereotypes, just up the road from the village of Si'umu.

After trying, unsuccessfully, to convince Mark, a cousin of my host, to dive from the lip of the gorge into the deepest pool, a major attraction of the park, we went and sat in a *fale* next to the women to smoke and talk about what else there was to see in Samoa. Near this *fale* a pipe and faucet rose out of the ground above a concrete platform. The tinned pop we had bought at the village store in Si'umu was gone and each of us filled our tins with water from this tap. The water was warm and sweet tasting and, I learned later, was not drawn from the nearby stream but from the reticulated water system which provides water to most of the villages on Upolu.

That evening I sat with my adoptive family, talking. They asked me about life in Canada, about what I hoped I would learn in Samoa. I told them how lucky I felt to have met their son while he was studying in Canada, and how proud I was to have been invited to come and live with his family during my fieldwork in Samoa. We talked about all the driving we had done that day, about how Julia, the second oldest son's wife, had never been to Togitogiga even though she was 30 years old and loved swimming in streams. We kidded Mark about being afraid to dive from the gorge and all promised to go back again, perhaps on the weekend, with spare clothes so that we could all go swimming. Throughout this discussion of diving, Mark was adamant about not diving. However, once it was suggested that we all go diving, he immediately agreed. Months later he would tell me that he had refused to dive from the gorge because his family had told him as a child that gorges such as Togitogiga are the favourite resting places of *aitu*, often malicious spirit beings who live throughout the islands. He would tell me that he had heard that a particularly vicious *aitu* lived at Togitogiga and that he was afraid of disturbing or angering her. However, when it was suggested that we all go diving, including myself, he agreed because he told me *palagi* — white people — were safe from attack by *aitu* and so he would be in no danger. An incident later in my stay, when an *aitu* threatened to kill a family I was visiting by causing the roof of their small wooden house to sway dangerously, shook his belief in my immunity to *aitu* attack and he admitted he was actually quite glad we never went back to Togitogiga.

It was several hours to dawn, and most of them I spent either curled on my hard bed or bending double out the doorway of my house, trying to vomit, to rid myself of the knot of pain and nausea that tore at my bowels and left me sweating and panicked. Slowly the village came awake, sounds of water running from outdoor taps, of window louvres being opened, of sleeping mats shaken against the side of trees and the now symphonic combination of crowing roosters and barking dogs coming from all sides of the house. The house I lived in had windows on all but one side, a concession in this European style bungalow to the open walled style of traditional *fale*. The combination of windows on three sides and the proximity of banks of short coconut palms and a bushy garden often made it difficult to determine where sound was coming from, an effect something like an envelope of sound which surrounds you.

I lay on the bed, still wrapped in a flannel sheet despite the now powerful sun which was warming the room and burning away the morning fog. I could hear the children of my household waking and moving through the house, their grandmother, Pai, calling them to hurry and bathe so they could eat their morning meal. I was frightened as I lay there, disoriented not only by the pain which made it difficult even to shift position on the bed, but also by the strangeness of the setting. I was literally nowhere, unable to get any bearings on the noises and the smells. I wanted to cry.

With a knock on the frame of the door which separated my sleeping area from the remainder of the house, and a gentle rattling of the beaded curtain that hung in the doorway, Pai, my host's wife and the woman who would become my mother during my stay in Samoa, came into the room carrying a tray with a pot of boiling water and a bottle of instant coffee. I didn't open my eyes for several minutes, and when I did she stood massively in the door looking down at me.

– Are you sick, she asked?

– Yes, in my stomach.

And she was gone, having set the tray of coffee on the floor. I'll be blunt. I had a momentary vision of her returning with some noxious herbal concoction, of chanting, dances, and National Geographic visions of long nights of hallucinations and strange evocative songs. However, I learned later in the day that after leaving the coffee Pai had gone to the Samoan *fale* behind my house where the senior members of my family lived, to inform them that Douglass was very sick. A hurried conference among the women came to some immediate practical decisions which included boiled eggs and heavily buttered toast. While they worked in the cookhouse, each of the five children living with us at the time came to my room and standing by the doorway, enquired after my health. A key moment came when ten-year-old Sene came and stood by the door.

– Did you get sick today, he asked me?

– I think so.

– A spook got you, that's right.

And he ran away laughing.

The village became noisier and noisier. The rusted and rattling water truck drove in to pick up several children to take them to school. Jerry, another cousin in this large extended family, who lived with his mother and brothers in the house directly beside mine, turned on his large radio and came outside dancing and singing a pop song by a Fijian superstar which seemed to be the only song anyone in Samoa would sing for months. Mark began driving the pigs into the area behind the cookhouse in order to select one to be sent to a wedding on the other side of the island.

Pai and Sina, one of her daughters-in-law, came back to my room about an hour after Pai had first seen me, carrying a larger tray on which lay several undercooked eggs and a plateful of buttered toast. Pai carried a large metal kettle which contained the weak heavily sweetened tea everyone drank throughout the day.

– We brought you something to eat, Sina told me. You should eat something if you are sick.

– Where are you really sick, Pai asked. Did you vomit or do something else?

– I've been vomiting all night but I don't think there is anything left.

– Then eat something now. Make things work so that things can move. Maybe later I will get some Samoan oil for you.

And they sat down, resting the tray at the foot of the bed, and watched me expectantly. The eggs, half cooked and slathered in beef drippings, were the cruellest tonic I had ever seen and as I pushed myself upright on the bed I wondered how I could convince these women that eating them would probably kill me. Pai held a cup of tea to me, told me to drink some and, as the lukewarm sweetness touched my lips I suddenly felt hungry, ravenous. I drank the tea hungrily and then made several small attempts at the eggs. As suddenly as it had come, the hunger was replaced by a wrenching cramp and I vomited noisily onto the floor. Silently, Sina and Pai helped me from the bed and took me down through the house to the indoor toilet where, after opening the door which was kept locked to keep the children away from the supply of tissue Pai kept, they left me leaning against the wall. Breathlessly I vomited over and over into the toilet. Exhausted, I fell asleep on the cool tile floor where I stayed until Mark came and shook me vigorously. Helping me to my feet, he wiped my face with the front of his t-shirt and then helped me back into bed. I slept again, waking late in the morning to the sound of a child singing as he pushed a crude contraption of sticks and buggy wheels back and forth in front of my house.

Julia came into the house calling my name. I was sitting up, changing into a cleaner shirt when she came into the room.

– Pai told us you were sick. Are you alright now?

– I feel terrible.

– What happened?

– I've been up most of the night throwing up and now I have a headache you wouldn't believe.

– Did you eat something?

– Some eggs but they made me sick again. They wouldn't stay down.

– You need to eat something else then. You need food if you've been vomiting all night.

She left and returned several minutes later with a dish of cold tinned spaghetti. She set it on my desk and then sat on the spare chair.

– We did too much yesterday. You drove too much. That's probably what made you sick. We should have stayed home longer. Maybe next time we won't go as far. You haven't been here very long.

– Jesus, Julia, you've lived in Canada. We drive that far almost every day.

– I know, but this is different, this is Samoa now and you should take it easy. Sonny shouldn't have let you drive.

– Well, I don't think I'll be driving for a while. I don't even think I'll be walking anywhere.

The spaghetti went down easily, only because I was able to swallow it quickly without chewing it. For the time being it also stayed down and after finishing it I sat back on the bed and tried to will my headache to subside. It didn't but I was still able to sleep again, waking in the afternoon only to begin vomiting again. Exhausted I sat in the door of my house watching the younger children going off to play rugby in a nearby village.

People I would later come to know well, women from neighbouring houses and some of their older sons, drifted by the house, stopping to enquire of my sick stomach. One woman came up to me while I had my eyes closed against the pain in my head and lay a small bunch of aromatic flowers in my hand. As I turned to thank her, another wave of nausea hit me and I vomited unceremoniously all over her lap. She took the flowers and set them beside me, then wiped at the corners of my mouth with her lavalava and whispered what I later learned was "well done, that vomiting."

Afternoon turned to evening, the shortest time of day in Samoa as the sun goes down so quickly dusk is over almost before you notice it has begun. I slept on and off through until nightfall, waking occasionally to go to the bathroom to try to vomit again. On one of these visits, Pai stopped me in the hall and asked if my bowels were working. They hadn't and I told her so.

– They will, she told me, then you will be alright.

Sina brought me some dinner sometime after seven, a plate of boiled taro and heated tinned mackerel but its appearance made even toying with eating it impossible. I asked her for some more tea and climbed back onto my bed. Several more people came by my windows as I lay there, asking how I was feeling and then leaving. A bell tolled in the next village and from each of the houses in my compound came the sound of evening prayers, a soft murmured sound punctuated by slow easy singing. It was now early evening and the *sā* had begun, a period of evening prayer when families gather around a lantern or a quietly flickering tv screen and the lively village noise subsides into a combination of softly sung hymns and the slow recitation of passages from the Bible.

Sonny, my host's oldest son, came to visit me later that night after the children had paid yet another enquiring visit. He brought me some cocoa, a thick sweet concoction of boiled ground cocoa and sugar, and a carton of cigarettes. He asked me what had happened, what I had been doing all day, how I felt. He asked me if I knew what was wrong and offered several possible answers. On our way back from Togitogiga we had stopped at a new bar/resort which was under construction by a retired American couple. We had sat in the nearly completed outdoor bar and had several local beers, together with a large platter of spicy fried octopus. Sonny wondered if maybe the beer had made me sick since it is so much stronger than Canadian beer. He then raised the question of driving again, wondering if I had perhaps driven too much for my first days in Samoa. Finally, he asked me about water. Had I drunk the water at Togitogiga, the water from the tap. I had and I told him, noting that at the time I was struck by how warm and sweet the water had tasted.

– I'm glad it was the water then. I wondered if maybe you didn't like Samoa or maybe Samoa wasn't going to like you but if it was the water then we know now.

He told me that the piped water I had drunk was not taken from the stream but from the island's reticulated water system. While stream water was usually very safe, he knew that *palagi* sometimes had problems with the local tap water. He explained to me that, historically, villages in Samoa were located away from the shore up the lower slopes of the ridge of volcanic mountains from which the islands are formed. They were also located within easy distance of the many small streams and rivers which cross the island. The reticulated water system, based on reservoirs high in the mountain ridge, was initially designed to serve the capital area of Apia and was being gradually extended to cover the entire island. Many Samoans feel the new piped water system is less safe than the older system of drawing water from nearby streams, in part because they doubt the Department of Public Works is sufficiently competent to ensure the sources are kept clear of detritus and contaminants, traditionally the practical and moral responsibility of villages along streams. It is not uncommon to find piped villages where the reservoir water is used solely for bathing and washing clothes, while drinking and cooking water is drawn in buckets from streams or stored in cisterns. He also told me that since I had arrived, Pai had been boiling all the water I had been drinking, always making certain there were several pitchers of chilled boiled water in the refrigerator in my house. A previous family guest, a student from England, had used tap water and had become violently ill for several days.

– Pai was worried you were unhappy here, that maybe you were too sad being away from Canada and that was making you sick but I should tell her it was the water at Togitogiga. That's what made you sick. You should drink the water Pai makes for you instead.

My panic was suddenly replaced by a sense of embarrassment, of guilt. Before leaving Canada for Samoa I had sought medical advice about adjusting to living and eating in Samoa. The only formal advice given to me was to force myself to drink the local water, to allow myself to become sick so that my body would adjust to the unfamiliar waterborne organisms. I was told it would likely be horrific and painful but that it was the quickest and simplest way to deal with the most common of travellers' complaints. I had said nothing on my arrival, in part fearing that raising the subject would insult my hosts. And so, from the moment I had arrived I had used the tap water, taking no more precautions than, occasionally, to pick a stray piece of leaf from my glass.

In doing that, I had not taken into account what my illness when it arrived would mean to the people around me. Sonny explained that Pai had spent part of the day consulting with two village *fofō* [healers] about how to help me get over my sadness, and that both had told her that if I was sick because I was sad, there would be no solution other than my going home. Everyone in my household compound had made a special point of visiting me, although only briefly, to ask after my stomach and to make me feel welcome. Sina had been berated by her father-in-law for failing to prepare my food properly. The children were threatened with a beating if they made any noise and disturbed me while I was unhappy. They were told to move slowly and quietly, to avoid running or talking loudly near my house. Henry, the youngest son in the family, even went so far as to push the family pickup truck almost a quarter mile away from the house before starting it in the morning, while local teenage boys chased village dogs away from the house to prevent their barking disturbing me. More disturbing for me was discovering that several people, including my host's elderly brother, were fined for failing to keep quiet during my illness.

There was another knock at my door and Sei'a, Sonny's father and the paramount political chief of both this village and the overall political district, came into my room. Behind him four boys stood holding a small wooden desk which still smelled of fresh varnish.

– Doug, you are having some cocoa. That's good. You will be able to sleep then. I asked Ioane to make you a desk for your studying. The boys can put it in here for you. You will be able to work there by the window.

Sei'a's presence added to my embarrassment, mostly because I had very quickly come to blame myself not only for my illness but also for the distress the family had experienced throughout the day. As the boys manouvered the desk in under the window, I mumbled thanks and explained that

I was beginning to feel much better. To punctuate this I drank deeply from the mug of tepid cocoa.

– We don't need to disturb you but Ioane wanted to bring you your desk as a gift to welcome you to the family. But there has been too much noise today already.

Sei'a spoke sharply to the boys, in Samoan, and they quickly placed the desk beneath the window and backed out of the room. I watched them, vaguely, not saying a word because I was afraid if I opened my mouth I would vomit once again.

Sei'a wished me a good night and pushed the boys from the house, stopping to remind Sonny that he shouldn't stay long and keep me talking. Sonny left a few minutes later.

When I woke the following morning, after a restful but often disturbed night's sleep, the absence of my earlier panic, combined with the course of anti-biotics brought with me from Canada, which I had begun the night before, made the still insistent pain and nausea more manageable. As the sun melted away the fog from the mangrove, I began to unpack my suitcases and tally up the effects of arriving on my peace of mind. The slow stirring of the village in those early moments of morning would always amaze me during my times in Samoa, and this one was doubly amazing because on one side of my house, facing the rising sun, the sky was sharpening into bright blue while on the other, away from sun, a light rain fell from a dark band of clouds caught for a moment between the sun and the mountains.

Sene, my ten-year-old little brother, came into my room and sat on the edge of the bed while I went through my clothes and books and papers.

– You have too many clothes.

– I know.

– Are you still sick today?

– I'm better. I even ate some bread from the cookhouse when I got up.

– Sei'a says maybe you are angry because Samoa is so strange and noisy.

– No, Sene, I think it was the water at Togitogiga that did it. *Palagi* have very weak stomachs.

– I had to sleep on Sei'a's bed yesterday. There was a monster in the *fale* who was trying to eat me.

– Did you see it?

– It came from over by the stream and walked around the *fale* for a long time calling me, saying Sene, it is time for school now. But I knew it was only a monster because it was still too dark to go to school. I think it wanted to eat me so I stayed on Sei'a's bed so that it would go away.

– Did it go away then?

– I think so. Pai told me she heard it before but that maybe it is only lost and couldn't find the stream again. Sometimes monsters get lost and then they wander around looking for strange people to eat. But maybe they won't eat *palagi*.

– If I see one, Sene, I'll go and sleep on Sei'a's bed with you.

– Do you like Samoa?

– Yes, very much.

– Then maybe you won't have to be angry anymore.

Throughout the next several days, as I risked leaving my house and walking about the village with Julia as my attentive guide, people who would later come to be intimate friends but who were, in those first weeks, absolute strangers by my cautious standards, would ask after my stomach and bowels and my happiness. They would question me closely about what I was now doing, with whom I was speaking, where I planned to visit. And they would, almost all of them, offer me both a diagnosis and an apology for Samoa making me sad and sick.

Embedded in these two days, in these first tentative and, at times, odd conversations, were the keys to everything I would ever learn about the body in Samoa. I saw none of this at the time. I did not notice the seriousness of Sene's joking about a spook nor did I fully understand why everyone in the village seemed to want to come to take a look at the sweating, nauseous *palagi* curled up on his bed. Julia's comments about the driving were meaningless and Pai's persistent enquiries about the condition of my bowels embarrassed but did not enlighten me. Had I understood Elizabeth's congratulations on my ill timed vomiting, it would have struck me as macabre rather than supportive.

Illness and blame, the play of responsibility, concern, interpretation and discipline, the way the people who would come to be my family and friends during my stay in Samoa deployed their understandings around the puzzle of my shivering body, all of this combined to push me beyond the limits of a flesh I thought I knew so intimately, toward a different kind of puzzle, one which made me begin to question, slowly and tentatively, the way bodies themselves are made to move in the world, and the way moving bodies make the world they occupy. Those questions are what this text explores, questions whose answers were there in the confusion of my first several days in Samoa, in the way my body was being remade by the circumstances and practices of the bodies around me.

Chapter 2

The Body in Question and the Question of the Body: Finding and Knowing Bodies in the Social Field

In a knot of eight crossings, which is about the average size knot, there are 256 different "over-and-under" arrangements possible... Make only one change in this "over-and-under" sequence and either an entirely different knot is made or no knot at all may result.

The Ashley Book of Knots

Every man takes the limits of his own field of vision for the limits of the world.

Schopenhauer in "Studies In Pessimism"

I recall, and will always remember, the shock of first seeing a palm tree at night, rising in the dark as cool and slim as a ghost. And what nights, bigger than imagining: black and gusty and enormous, disordered and wild with stars. On such a night, after a long day of thunderous, dolorous storms, I borrowed a bike from a neighbour in the village of Vaimoso, Samoa,[1] where I would live for more than a year, and rode ponderously up the village road toward the one small shop that sold American cigarettes. Set back from the road, thatched open walled houses and cottage-like bungalows were, in the brilliance of incandescent light against the darkness of a moonless Pacific night, a slide show of tableaux: family scenes and sleeping children, women hanging mosquito nets over mats or sitting in quiet circles talking and drinking cocoa, and clusters of teenage boys sitting just on the fringe of the web of light, laughing. Occasionally someone would call to me on the road, ask where I was going or simply wish me a goodnight.

To reach the store, I had to pass over a bridge that crosses the often muddy stream that splits the village of Vaimoso down its centre. Bridges in Samoa are special places, because rivers and streams are popular throughways for *aitu* [often malicious spirit beings], who travel from the

13

sky forest on the range of mountains which divide the main island of Upolu, to the sea. The streams and rivers become a nightly concourse of moving spirits. Rivers in Samoa are always places of respect and caution. At night they become places of real, sometimes fatal danger.

As I approached the bridge, I climbed down from my bike and pushed it cautiously along the road, looking up and down the Gasegase Stream as if looking both ways before crossing a busy street. The skin on the back of my neck and on my hands, holding the gripless rusted handlebar, began to prickle and moisten. I could feel the subtle grip of anxiety deepen my breathing, and my face tensed into an attentive pucker.

And then I was on the bridge and then I was over it, walking quickly several metres away before I climbed back on my bike and pedalled along to the store, and a soul soothing Camel.

I went to Samoa with a specific question in mind: how and why do Samoans choose between the two forms of healing available to them? However, the more I learned about the different aspects of illness and cure, the more often I had to shift my focus, and reexamine the implications of the questions I was asking. The seemingly simple issue of decision making processes, a question that remains central to the kind of research I continue to do in Samoa, and other Pacific societies, as well as locally in Canada, became entangled in a different set of questions, revolving around the process by which a person, or the persons around them, make the decision that he or she is, indeed, sick. This set of questions led me to realize that to understand that set of practices, I first needed to begin to understand how the body is itself understood, before it can be understood as a sickened thing. This realization compelled me to recognize that to get at illness as one special case of body practice, I first needed an analytic frame that would allow me to understand what it means to have, and to be, a body at all. This search for such an analytic frame led me to begin disassembling the nature of the sick body in Samoan culture, asking what was being done, where and why and how, by whom, and according to what rules. From this I extended my focus to questions of how the body is understood and treated as a reliable and predictable locus of social knowledge and practical action, that is, the process of thinking about and enacting a meaningful body that I call embodiment: the combination, in practice, of organic sensations and form, cultural ideals and meanings, and the particular lived experience of individual bodies, on which and through which the meaning and effect of the body are enacted as an ongoing, fluid, process.

The body poses a fundamental puzzle for anthropology because it is simultaneously, the most obvious object in the social world, and the most elusive. The argument I will make in what follows is that the body is a conundrum in that it is always present, an unavoidable object, and always changing, always being invented and reinvented. It is elusive and persistent, quietly constant and constantly disquieting, both a site of social action and one of its causes. Grasping the body analytically is difficult precisely because its presence is the most taken-for-granted aspect of sociality, rendering transparent the web of enactments through which people manage to engage the world and their bodies in it.

In those brief seconds as I moved toward, then over, and then away from the bridge over the Gasegase Stream, my body collided with my expectations in a mosaic of biology and memory and imagination, in an enactment both of my body and of the world with my body in it. The sweat on my palms, and the prickling skin on the back of my neck, were diacritics of an ongoing and reciprocal dialogue between what the body is as a thing in the universe, and what the body is as a meaningful project we are all engaged in, from that point of consciousness when we recognize where our body ends, and where the world begins. The body is a process through which we negotiate and manipulate that boundary, giving meaning and form to the thing we are in the world. It is a process through which that boundary between being in the world, and the world itself, shifts and vibrates with intention and attention. Through this we embody the world by embodying our self in it.

In this text I will advance an outline of embodiment in Samoa, by focussing on the body as an ongoing process, rather than simply an artifact of culture. Embodiment is a process that is continuous, shifting, and never complete, because the body is not only something we "do to," but also something we "do." That is to say, in doing something to the body, we are not only acting on an object, we are also enacting the body itself. The study of embodiment can open a window into this aspect of culture, making it possible to see culture constituted in the way people walk or play, in the way people treat illness, or initiate their young with scarring and ritual. A model of embodiment will allow us to move beyond the grammar of bodies as solely objects acted upon, toward an understanding of how bodies themselves are created in everyday social action, and in being created, create the very ground on which social action is possible. Such an understanding can locate health and health making practices squarely in a context which links this specific issue to both the largest and smallest details of being a good and proper body in a good and proper world.

The Body Objected To: Theoretical Approaches to The Body

The good and proper body, a phrase I am borrowing from the work of the neo-Freudian linguist and psychoanalyst, Julia Kristeva, is not simply a thing of blood and bile and bone. The phrase, which I will use often throughout this book, is meant to evoke a complex of connections which site the body as a living practice, as something which is always being created, always only imminent in the social field. That social field, like the bodies in it, is conditioned by historical contingency and a persistent philosophical engagement between individuals, their communities, the structures and institutions within which and through which they live and concerns and considerations for appropriate social and physical presence. That is, the body as I am using the concept here, is an ongoing process of moral accountability in which well-being, propriety, and local instantiations of righteousness conjoin in the practice of culture as a kind of embodied and entailed piety. The religious imagery is appropriate as the body I am talking about is always an engagement with the world in which reflection, obeisance and supplication, and the twin practices of submission and transgression enact an ordered, though not necessarily orderly, world.

Bodies, as organic phenomena, may be said to have an independent existence, independent, that is, of consciousness. Such existence, like that of plants, or moss stains on a rock, is the meanest form of existence, an existence with no being. The body I am interested in is the body attended to, that is, the body seen, interpreted, and experienced. This process of attention is the pre-objective state of subjectivity, and it determines how distinctions between things are enacted. Attention is pre-objective because it "exists" prior to the object being attended to having any meaning at all. It is the ground for meaning, and therefore, objectification [Csordas 1990]. Attention both constitutes meaningful objects, and is a function of the ongoing constitution of the social field as something in which meaningful objects may exist. It is a relationship between things, and the meanings of things, in the sense that attention is a set of anticipations about what, in the world, can be seen. Attention is the basic code which determines what can and cannot be an object, and what can and cannot be observed. The enacted body is not the only "object" to which attention is turned, but it is the most complex, since the meaningful body is both a thing and a consciousness of a thing. That is, it is complicit in the attention to which it is subjected. The body, therefore, can never be completely separated from the manner in which it is observed and made meaningful, because the body, as a thing which is conscious of itself, is always engaged in making itself observable, something which can and should be attended to. By doing anything with the body, we engage the gaze of others in a mutual, circular, reciprocal process of being seen by making our selves, as embodied and embodying projects, visible and sensible. We become what we intend others to see by attending to what can be seen in others, a relationship of mutual accountability and the moral ordering of embodied presence.

Most anthropological approaches to the body have failed to recover from the field of social action the processes through which the body is, in practice, enacted in the world as a moral praxis. In general, such studies of the cultured body are a kind of encyclopedia of effects, a study of how culture is inscribed on the body. They assume a body prior to culture, which is manipulated, manoeuvred, and interpreted through a cultural lens. I want to explore some of these approaches briefly, to show how what I am proposing builds on, and departs, from what these approaches have accomplished. However, this review cannot even begin to do justice to the proliferation of literature on the body since Marcel Mauss's *Techniques of the Body* first outlined an anthropology of the body nearly 60 years ago [Synnott 1993]. In recent years, but especially since the 1977 publication of Blacking's edited volume, *The Anthropology of the Body*, the depth and range of literature in the social sciences and humanities which focusses, either explicitly or implicitly, on the body, has grown so dramatically that it is not unreasonable to speak of the anthropology of the body as an emerging sub-discipline in its own right. My goal here is not a review but a brief travelogue through the kinds of ideas and issues which inform my own formulation of the body in Samoa that I am presenting here.

Since the early 1980's several general discussions of the body, framed around issues of illness, health, and ethnopsychiatry, have appeared [Glassner 1988; Stigler, Schweder and Herdt 1990; Helman 1990,1991; Featherstone, Hepworth and Turner 1991; Feierman and Janzen 1992; Lindenbaum and Lock 1993; Kunitz 1993; Good 1994]. Along with these general texts, there has been what Synnott [1993:228] refers to as a "veritable cascade" of books on special topics:

- pleasure [Ferguson 1990; Parker 1991; Tiger 1992];
- pain [Scary 1985; Morris 1991; DelVechhio-Good, Brodwin, Good and Kleinman 1992];
- sex and sexuality [Herdt 1982, 1984; Gallagher and Laquer 1987; Butler 1990, 1993];
- gender, gender ambiguity and body representations [Williams 1986; Hanna 1988; Clatterbaugh 1990; Epstein and Straub 1991; Roscoe 1991; Fuss 1991; Silverman 1992; Garber 1992; Herdt 1994];
- the discovery of the invisible interior of the body in Western art and medicine and its effect on the practice of body and self knowledge [Stafford 1991];
- emotions and the somaticization of cultural categories [Lutz 1988];
- AIDS[2] and its effect on modern bio-social body politics [Bateson and Goldsby 1988; Crimp 1988; Sontag 1989; Herdt and Lindenbaum 1992; Farmer 1992];

- sexualized bodies and national identity [Mosse 1985; Theweleit 1987, 1989; Parker, Russo, Sommer and Yaeger 1992];
- tattooing [Sanders 1989; Mascia-Lees and Sharpe 1992; Gell 1993]
- an increasing number of culturally specific ethnographic studies which use the body as the ground of enquiry— Papua New Guinea [Battaglia 1990; Weiner 1988,1991; Gillison 1993; Lewis 1980; Frankel 1989]; Mexico [Finkler 1991]; Belau [Parmentier 1987]; Southern Africa [Comaroff 1985]; India [Alter 1993]; China [Zito and Barlow 1994]; North America [Martin 1987]; Ireland [1991]; Brazil [Parker 1991]; Australia (Pintupi) [Myers 1991] and The Phillipines (Ilongot) [Rosaldo, M. 1980; Rosaldo, R. 1980] to name but only a few.

As this partial list of body oriented studies suggests, the problem of the body as a theoretical object, returns and returns, in Coleridge's phrase, in "obstinate resurrection." What separates most of these texts from what I am proposing here, however, is the tendency of most body studies to focus on specific kinds of bodies, or exotic instances of body practice, such as ritual, healing, or gender. In contrast, the model of the body in Samoa I will explore here seeks to demonstrate the linkages between the most trivial and the most exotic forms of body practice in the constitution of culture and action.

Sickness and Social Bodies

More than almost any other subject in the social sciences, the study of human suffering has vexed and engaged thinkers and theorists for decades. I want to consider here three very general approaches this area of thinking has explored because I feel that, taken together, these perspectives represent the best that medical anthropology and sociology have offered, and open the greatest number of possibilities to which an embodied analysis of culture and society can contribute.

David Mechanic [1974, 1978], for example, took up the challenge of Parsons's notion of the "sick role." From Mechanic's perspective, illness involves the transfer of the person into a special state of being, distinctive from normal social roles, into what Susan Sontag [1978] calls the "kingdom of the sick." Sick role theory explores the processes through which a person is recognized as sick, is granted new status as a sick person, and details the obligations and privileges this new role entails, not only for the sick person, but for the people around him or her.

This idea of spaces of illness [Good 1994] advances the study of bodies and persons, because it opens illness to scrutiny as a set of practices.

In recognizing the play of power and resistance, and of privilege and obligation, in the process of being ill and becoming well, sick role theory provides fundamental insights into the question of how the body is deployed as a strategy in social relations. By analyzing both illness and wellness as states or conditions negotiated over, sick role theory links the experience of the body to questions of agency and action, and exposes the body as a practice rather than only a thing practised upon.

However, there is also a fundamental limitation to the sick role approach. By virtue of its focus on roles, the body is conceived of as a thing reacted to, a not-me object [Petrunik and Shearing 1988; Winnicot 1986]. This confines our ability to see the body in action because it elides completely the question of how an actor comes to see his or her body as "other." By what practice does the body become super-corporeal, something the person acts on rather than something the person acts with. That is, the body in this model is a thing done to, is already there in the world waiting to be acted upon, missing entirely the question of how the body, in practice, comes to have a meaningful presence, and how this presence is maintained.

Brody [1987] in his work on how the stories we tell about illness help constitute the illness experience, Kleinman [1980] in his analysis of how beliefs are a fundamental aspect of the construction and experience of illness, and Helman [1991, 1990] in his writings on the cultural aspects of illness experience, have attempted to move beyond the reifying limitations of the sick role model by building on the importance of intersubjective negotiation in understanding the process of illness and health. These authors focus on the question of illness and the body, and their relationship to the construction of self knowledge. They argue that illness is often about negotiations and arbitrations through which a person's sense of self is generated, justified, and legitimated. They recognize that the somatic phenomenon of illness cannot be disengaged from the somatizing effects of culture and they call into question the comforts of a universal biological body by arguing that culture restricts how the body can be experienced, while at the same recognizing, as Boddy reminds us, that "[however] cultural and mindful bodies may be, to the extent that they are singular entitities, they are singular processes" [1998:252].[3]

Such insights begin to locate the body at the nexus between culture and self awareness, but they do so by proposing a kind of fundamentally innocent, universal body onto which the trauma of illness as a cultural phenomenon is mapped. As far as it goes, this approach is central to our understanding of the body as a culturally centred, enacted, epistemological phenomenon but even with these refinements, the body remains a thing acted upon, a kind of ur-object around which culture is practised. The body is objectively naive, rather than an exquisite and calculated practice.

Finally, Turshen's [1984, 1991] work on public health and political power in rural Africa, as well as other developments in Critical Medical Anthropology [Baer and Singer 1997] have advanced the study of the body. Work such as Turner [1984], on the sociology of power in illness and healing in Britain, and Harkin's [1994] recent work on the constitution of power, personhood and illness among the Heiltsuk people of the Central British Columbia coast, argue that illness, in its definition, epidemiology and practice, cannot be isolated from structures of power. Building on Foucault's [1973] notion that the "clinical gaze" is a political process, and not only a scientific or curative one, these authors connect illness and the body to larger processes of political authority, domination, and surveillance. They expose the micro-physics of motivation which affect how the body is known, knowable, and controlled, by drawing attention to larger political issues of who defines illness and health, who has the power to enforce rules of proper body practice, and how resistance, through the use of illness and the body, can be linked to larger social practices of power and authority.

Taken together, these accomplishments in medical anthropological theory provide fertile prospects for developing increasingly sophisticated understandings of how bodies are invented and manipulated in social action. They also ignore what, for me, remains a fundamental question. While recognizing that in illness practice, as with all other body practices, there is an object, "a body," out there in the social field to be acted upon, the problem of how that "object" is constituted and maintained is never addressed. Rather, each of these approaches begins with the assumption of a fundamental and universal body, which cultures act upon, without raising the vexing question of how anyone ever comes to apprehend the body at all. This is not simply a question of self awareness, or of the psychology of body image and body sensation.[4] Sensations occur, after all, independently of our "recognizing" them. My concern is not with whether bodies exist as organic processes, but with how we come to attach meaning to these processes. What these and other medical anthropological models have not yet addressed is the question of how the body comes to be meaningful at all.

The field of ethno-medicine [for example Nichter 1992; Frankel and Lewis 1989] has taken up the challenge of this limitation in medical anthropology by exploring how cultural systems of embodiment constitute bodies differently, breaking through the restriction of a universal body by arguing that bodies need to be understood as culturally distinctive, an insight which has informed the development of the ideas I explore here. By taking ethnobiologies seriously and granting them the same epistemological and practical weight often automatically granted to "scientific" biology, these authors raise questions about the nature of body experience by arguing that it is not simply a question of different cultures having different understandings of body processes. Rather, different cultures might have different bodies altogether. The *to'ala*, or stomach-heart, of Samoan anatomy, while not appearing in any scientific biology text, must, according to the arguments advanced by those working in the field of ethnomedicine, be recognized as a real organ for those who experience its existence, and the distress it can produce. This raises the question of how bodies are constituted as meaningful things more fully than conventional medical anthropology and medical sociology, without denying the insights and advances these models have provided. More than simply adding new data to the question of how bodies and illnesses are done, ethnomedical research has expanded the scope of questions medical anthropology can ask by problematizing the very nature of the body itself.

Art, Artifice and the Inscribed Body

One the most prominent places occupied by body studies in general anthropology has been the study and analysis of body modification practices in societies around the world. These studies examine such diverse practices as body painting, tattooing, circumcision and other forms of altering surgery, costume, and the many other kinds of attachments and alterations to which the body is subjected. They offer a more complete picture of how the body can be deployed and manipulated as a social process.

Whether O'Hanlan's [1989] analysis of body decoration in Papua New Guinea, Knauft's [1989] discussion of the poetics of body marking throughout Melanesia, or Herdt's [1982] edited volume on the embodying effects of initiation surgery on young boys in Papua New Guinea, the study of body modification has been one of anthropology's most substantial contributions to the opening up of a vigourous and critical understanding of the nature of the body in social space. Such studies recognize that the body is an important surface on which social action can be deployed and enacted. They also draw our attention to the fact that, in looking at how the surface of the body is modified by social action, it is necessary to relate these superficial alterations and expressions to the way the body is experienced and practised as a totality. Studies of body modification remind us that the body is not only surfaces, it is scents and smells and ways of moving; it is internal processes and webs of external connections which draw together all the fundamental processes of culture at the site of culture's most intimate expression; it is an active matrix of possibilities as much as it is a machine that eats and sleeps and hungers and hurts.

This has also been a deficiency in the anthropology of the body modification. Although body modification studies have long recognized and dealt with the question of the invention of the body, they have most often done so either implicitly or superficially. That is, body modification studies are about how the body is an active invention, since they deal with the questions of how the modification and experience of the body are inseparable, but they do so in the context of a model of the body as a singular, universal phenomenon. Like medical anthropology, and perhaps precisely because body modification studies combine biology and aesthetics, the question of how that canvas is arrived at is not directly addressed. The evidence of modification as actively creating the body, in the sense, for example, that nosebleeding of Gnau boys remakes their bodies as stronger and as male [Lewis 1980], is constrained by the theoretical limitations which posit a fundamental body onto which this transformation is a superficial overlay, theorizing body modification from the institutions of modification down onto the body rather than "theorize[ing these] institutions from the body up" [Frank 1991:49].

Relating bodies as artifacts of social action to the wider institutions within which bodies are deployed is important. However, the approach I have adopted in this text takes the focus on the body in a different direction, applying a model of observation and analysis that scrutinizes the totality of the body as ongoing and invented, rather than encompassing the body in some other form of social totality, of which the body is simply an object or, at best, an objective. In each of the attempts to theorize the body I have described above, the presence of the body as a meaningful thing has been treated, at worst, as completely unproblematic and, at best, as a simple artefact of the practices, whether diagnosis and healing or ritual modification, which have been applied to it. What is left to be explained is Mauss's recognition, over half a century ago, that the body is not an object at all, but "the condition for objectification" [cited in Deutsch 1993:11]

The Body as Histories Inside Histories

There is an area of study outside anthropology that has made significant contributions to what I see as the process of building a model of the social body. The development of a field of historical body study has begun to unravel the puzzle of the body, to which the preceding paragraphs have alluded.[5] Bodies have histories, not only in terms of beliefs or practices, but in terms of each individual body itself. That is the puzzle I am exploring. How are bodies enacted as particularized sets of practices which inexorably invent the very body itself, rather than simply revising how the body is understood, creating the particular body of a specific cultural moment, by the practices through which it is understood and employed?

Early attempts at body history, such as Gallagher and Lacquer's [1987] studies of the emergence of the modern sexualized body, begin from an assumption that there had been some fundamental shift in how the body is understood, a function in part of new knowledge, and in part, of new political power structures. Similarly, Martin's work on reproductive technologies [1987] focussed on the shifts which had occurred in the way bodies, as *a priori* objects, could be manipulated and constrained as a result of changes in the way the body was technically understood. More recent studies build on Foucault's assertion that the nature of the gaze turned on the body determines how that body is treated and manoeuvred in relationships of power [1973, 1979]. For example, Allen Feldman [1991] explores how, in the context of political disarray and civil war in Northern Ireland, the body is constantly reformulated and re-experienced in the political field such that individual experiences of the body are often the very engine which drives political action. His analysis of the process of embodiment in relation to the IRA prisoner's hunger strikes of the 1970's and 1980's argues for an understanding of political action in Northern Ireland in terms of the kinds of bodies the various antagonists have, whether the emotionless and insensitive body of the "hardman" or the machine body of the British Troops. Feldman argues that the civil war has created these kinds of bodies, and that once created, their existence perpetuates the war that has created them, since their existence has come to depend on that war. These kinds of bodies are derived from the history of the conflict. Through them, not only is the body historicized, but history is somaticised.

In another example, Duden [1991] describes the medical experiences of a group of women in 18th century Germany, and argues that the very bodies they had were different from the bodies we know today. Not only their knowledge, but the way they experienced menstruation as a heating up of the blood, made their bodies separate from modern German women's bodies. She challenges us to think about the organic body as something which is, itself, altered by the practices of embodiment through which it is understood and experienced. In effect, what Duden is suggesting is that we stop thinking in terms of differing medical or somatic models as ideas about the same basic thing, and begin to think in terms of distinctive bodies altogether. Her work argues that "Western" scientific medicine and biology are also ethnomedicine and ethnobiology, and that they should be treated analytically with the same critical rigour we bring to bear on those of other cultures and times. Her call for a rigorous effort to recapture what she calls the "lost bodies of the past" has been an important motivation in my own work, drawing me to understand that to get to this archaeology of previous forms of the body, it is first necessary to devise a method for excavating the present such as Martin [1994] who offers a suggestive method for doing an ethnography of the body in her historically and ethnographically informed analysis of the concept of immunity in the shaping of embodied health practice in the United States. Such a focus on embodiment as a concept engine, if you will, represents an approach to embodiment and social practice which complements the focus on everyday embodiment I pursue here. Taken together, these two approaches offer a way to instrumentalize the model of the body I am exploring in this book.

One contribution to the development of these methods is the work of Scheper-Hughes and Lock [1987], and of Lindenbaum and Lock [1993], on the social basis of lived bodies. In their 1987 paper, Scheper-Hughes and Lock argue that we need to think of the body as having a tripartite structure, that is

> (1) as a phenomenally experienced *individual body-self*; (2) as a *social body*, a natural symbol for thinking about relationships among nature, society and culture; and (3) as a *body-politic*, an artifact of social and political control [1987:6, emphasis in original].

They recognize that the body, in sickness and in health, is "a form of communication...through which nature, society and culture speak simultaneously" (31). It is their insight, as Frank [1991] notes, to synthesize the concurrent puzzles of being a body, having a body, and having a body that is done to, and to open the question of how medical anthropology can begin to address this conflation.

Lindenbaum and Lock take up this challenge in the introduction to their edited volume of conference papers, noting that a renewed critical vigour in the anthropology of the body can help us to understand

> how different practices change modes of knowing and conceptions of the self...by moving them to a new field site, at once familiar, but now conceptually different, since the body itself, with its insistent subjectivity, provokes us to inquire into the historical processes whereby biological and cultural phenomena are mutually determined [1993:xiv].

By exploring how different histories, and different moments in history, produce different bodies, not only ideologically, but also experientially, such an analytic strategy raises questions an embodied anthropology can begin to address.[6] A focus on historicity, and most importantly, on lived history as a quotidian process of embodied engagement in the world, is of fundamental importance to any method of embodied analysis because it begins to locate natural objects inside historical process both as causative and consequential components of those histories.[7]

The Body as Paradigm

Anthropology has been over-burdened in its history by the pursuit of an unified theory of social life and order, but the one thing anthropologists are guaranteed to disagree on is a working definition of culture. Indeed, it is the very richness of culture as an analytic frame which obstructs its fruitfulness as a focus of knowledge in anthropology. The points of connection which make up "cultures" are too various, too ill defined, and their salience as general principles is either immeasurable or constantly shifting in the histories and agenda of both the people observed and the people observing. Myth, politics, ritual, and superstructure and infrastructure, make up, both in the sense of being components of, and in the sense of inventing, cultures. It is not that culture is unknowable, but simply that what can be known about culture is never static, and not the same thing to all participants.

At the same time, however sophisticated our attempts to codify "culture" as an analytic focus, the act of analysis in terms of cultural wholes is itself an "enculturing act" which cannot move beyond the fundamental difficulty that the only culture anthropology knows is that culture which it invents within the frames of its theoretical orientations and its political, narrative, and even moral agenda [Abu-Lughod 1993]. The anthropology of culture struggles against the compelling problem that the enculturing gaze of the anthropological observer is teleological. Even those efforts to critique this effect [Marcus and Fisher 1986; Clifford and Marcus 1986] simply invert the problem by adding a different, ill-defined, totalizing, enculturing gaze which looks back at the anthropologist.

Recent work on the body has offered what I think is one solution to this theoretical puzzle, by proposing that we move our analytic gaze toward the most intimate process in human existence, the process by which we come to have meaningful, practical, socially effective bodies. Thomas Csordas has made the most substantial contribution to date, through his analysis of the principles of embodiment which underlie Christian Charismatic healing in America [Csordas 1994, 1993, 1990]. He argues that what is needed in anthropology is a fundamental paradigm shift away from the question of aggregates and collectivities, to a more basic ground of experience, the individual's presence in the world as a meaningful body. Combining phenomenology and Bourdieu's concept of habitus, Csordas argues that we need a new model of culture which locates the body, a historically and experientially specific body, as an important, if not the most important, site at which culture is enacted. He suggests that we need to understand culture not only in terms of what people believe, but in terms of how they do or believe anything about the world as an aspect of constituting their bodies. Csordas is arguing for a different model of existence which takes, as its fundamental problem, how any person comes, in the course of their organic existence, to understand how to live and move as a body in the world. Taking up that call is, at least in part, what this text endeavours to do.

Several recent attempts to develop this approach from an ethnographic ground have advanced the emergence of an embodied paradigm in interesting ways. Becker [1995] examines the practices of embodiment in the construction of Fijian social life in order to explore how structures and institutions form a conceptual and practical network through which Fijians are able to maintain a sense of ordered social presence. Through a startling and sophisticated analysis of survey data on ideal body image, Becker is able to demonstrate how embodied praxis in Fiji contrasts with the Western obsession with cultivating the body as an ideal object, and further and most intriguing for me, she argues for locating self as an ongoing practice for Fijians at a peculiar nexus where Fijians actively alienate themselves form their body as object in order to experience their body in a more sociocentric, communal frame.

The various authors in Lambek and Strathern, eds. [1998] chart a different, but equally compelling course in the collection of papers which explore the intricacies of embodied experience, self-awareness, and proper social identity or personhood. Apart from revitalizing comparative analysis both across cultural domains in a single society, and across cultural boundaries between societies, the papers in this volume demonstrate with ethnographic rigour and critical acumen the depth of knowledge and understanding of embodiment which lies just beneath the surface of much anthropological analysis. More importantly, they point toward the several directions research in this field must pursue, not the least of which is a re-theorizing of cognition, self-concept, and identity from an embodied perspective, a theme explored in even greater detail and depth in Lakoff and Johnson monumental review of Western philosophical traditions and the "problem of the body" [Lakoff and Johnson 1999].

Finally, though not exhaustively, Butler [1993] sets out a theoretical agenda which seeks to destabilize the normative effect of biology as an a priori category in approaching embodiment and social process. Arguing that bodies are things thought rather than simply things thought about, and drawing attention to the shifting conceptual ground on which biology is deployed not so much as a science but as a rhetorical strategy, she shows how any approach to embodiment must begin before the body. That is, she argues for a recognition that bodies are a consequence of practices of embodiment in which matter, in this instance bodies, made meaningful through political and cultural engagement, is matter made socially real.

My own ongoing work seeks to develop these ideas further through the analysis of such processes as the enactment of homosexually aroused bodies by cognitively and socially heterosexual male prostitutes, and the ways in which elderly women resist the negations of the elderly female body offered them by medical science by deploying their bodies as energetic, healthy, sexual, and socially important. A third analysis looks at the ways good and proper bodies are manifest in the contentions between a mainstream urban gay neighbourhood, and two contiguous neighbourhoods — one predominantly Afro-carribean and the other a commercial street sex neighbourhood. In each instance, I am pursuing ways in which an embodied approach can be theorized and engaged as a fulsome model for social analysis and critique.

No review of work on the body as a social process, to borrow Turner's phrase, can be complete. My purpose in this short summary is simply to draw a sketch of the analytic landscape within which studies of the body and of the various manifestations of body practice I am referring to here as embodiment. The study of the body, like social bodies themselves, remains a work in progress. But what each of these various approaches illuminate is a need to reconfigure the anthropological gaze in the direction of a more intimate ground on which no thing, especially the body, can be taken for granted. Such a turn brings anthropologies holism closer to fruition, I suggest, by asking a different set of questions about the connections between being in the world, being of the world, and being the world itself, all central aspects of an embodied perspective which I am applying here.

Recovering the Samoan Body: Prospectus and Agenda

In *Natural Symbols*, [1970] Mary Douglas writes of the two bodies, of the self, and of society, and argues that "sometimes they are so near as to be almost merged [and] sometimes they are far apart. *The tension between them allows the elaboration of meaning*" [1970:112, emphasis added]. Meaning is at the heart of the acts of embodiment this text will explore: meaning as a process of constituting the world, as an artifact of action, and as the foundation of how bodies are made. The thoughtful body, the body upon which I focus here, is the body imagined into existence by attention and interpretation and practice. It is not a body mapped on top of some organic body, whether genital or gustatory or respiratory, although the thoughtful body can never be isolated from these organic realities. Instead, the thoughtful body is the account given of those features of the organic body which, through the lived history of being a body, each person enacts, as a fundamental ground of social action. The thoughtful body is the "real," lived, meaningful body. What I am proposing is a shift in body studies from the question of managing bodies as "biological, material entit[ies]" [Csordas 1993:135] to a focus on the body as an ongoing practice of constitution in which semantic information [models, concepts, ideals] is not separated from episodic information [particular experiences, particular lived bodies], that is, as "an indeterminate methodological field defined by perceptual experience and the mode of presence and engagement in the world" [Csordas 1993:135]. Not only are "bodies good to think," to revitalize an observation of Levi-Strauss's, they are also necessary to think. The primary issue my discussion in this text raises is the puzzle that, without bodies there is no culture and that without culture, there are no bodies.

A student once responded to a lecture on the nature of culture with the comment that "culture is the process of creating culture." To his comment I would add the codicil that the body, as well, is about creating a body. The tautology is unavoidable. The argument I am making here directs our attention to the fundamental issue of the constructedness of the world and of our presence in it.[8]

Study of the thoughtful body can be useful in the continuing revitalization of the concept of culture in anthropology, in the same way as the practice of embodiment is central to the ongoing vitalization of culture as a lived experience. The thoughtful body focusses attention on culture as the constitution and deployment of meaningful things in constituted, meaningful space. The move I am proposing involves a shift from an anthropology of the done to an anthropology of doing, by recognizing that the done, that is culture as retrospection, is better understood as something we are always doing, culture as prospective, as the generation of possibility. It entails a recognition that being and experience, conjoined as they are in the constitution of this ongoing, projective, culture process, are always decentred, transient, and cumulative. Lived experience and culture are not distinguishable. Lived experience does not "happen" inside of culture, and culture is not the simple coral-like accumulations of lived experience. Culture is a verb, it is active and participatory, and an emergent property of the engagement between the process of generating meaning, the practices of embodiment, and the relationships of unique individuals in socially meaningful space. This view of culture and the body emphasizes the need to shift our focus away from the notion of body knowledge as a repertoire available to actors by redefining the body as a generative practice rather than a reactive one. That is, the body is a practice which needs to be seen as an indivisible fraction of the constitution of culture itself.

To emphasize the importance of this aspect of the study of embodiment, the practices and habits I will talk about in the chapters to follow should be understood as no more exotic than what you or I did this morning when we washed and dressed and went about our various jobs. To reinforce this ordinariness I have chosen the aspects of Samoan bodies I will explore explicitly for their mundane, quotidian quality. This is to ensure that what I have to say about Samoan embodiment is not construed as strange, and to convey to you that the process of embodiment is present in every act. Indeed, the question of where to look for insight into embodiment is moot. Look anywhere, since in every moment of every act, the practice of embodiment is necessarily and always present. Whether the elaborate manipulations of a circumcision ritual in the Highlands of Papua New Guinea or the joyful dance of a twelve-year-old boy around the stalls of the new market in Apia, Samoa, on finding a shiny dollar coin among the debris of taro leaves and cigarettes, acting in the world in any capacity is an act of embodiment, and deserves close and careful scrutiny and consideration.

The choice of sites of body enactment on which the following chapters are based is also framed by the kinds of understandings I came to have about the precepts and concerns Samoans bring to bear on their everyday affairs. Although I will develop these ideas more fully in the next chapter, I want to note that my selection, while guided by a desire for simplicity, and an avoidance of the exotic, was nonetheless affected by three fundamental concerns — about dignity, humility, and strength — which pervade all social action in Samoa. In choosing aspects of embodiment to discuss in this text, I have done so with an eye to demonstrating how these three key themes underlie all body practices for Samoans. In tracing the outlines of how the body is enacted in Samoa, I will show how these three concerns form the experiential ground on which Samoans live in, and through their bodies.

An issue I will not address in detail in these chapters is that of sexing and gender. Gender and sexing in Samoa is a subject of great complexity, and is an issue I continue to work on, in ongoing research on third gendered males in the Pacific. I feel the study of "gendering the world" [vis Abu-Lughod 1993] is an area to which a comprehensive model of embodiment can make a significant contribution, and Mageo [1998] is a recent attempt, though from a perspective different than mine, to address this issue in Samoa. I want to stress, as Mageo does, that the continuing understanding of Samoan sociality demands a critical understanding of the vexatious and apparently fragmenting practices of sexing and gendering in Samoa. At the same time, as I will argue at several points, there is an ambiguity and transience to Samoan gender such that talking about males and females as fixed states with rigidly constrained natures and characters is misleading. That ambiguity and transience posed a fundamental problem which troubled me during my times in Samoa. It is a simple problem but one which tested my ability to read the bodies of the people around me. Stated simply:

How does a North American man reconcile an engendered order where sex with a biological male is not a homosexual act?

Samoa, like elsewhere in Polynesia, has an institutionalized non-male gender role, enacted by bearers of biologically male bodies. The *fa'afafine*, translating as approximately "of the way of women," are characteristically flamboyant, superficially female and participate in all aspects of Samoan life. They vary, most distinctively when comparing the often outrageous *fa'afafine* who live and work in Apia, Samoa's one town with those who live in the outer villages, who tend to be more demure. Socialization into *fa'afafine* status can be initiated by a parent, usually the mother, or can be chosen by the individual themselves. While this is changing, currently most *fa'afafine* marry, or plan to marry. In their own characterization of themselves, *fa'afafine* are not simply effeminized men but a sex unto themselves. The are often the butts of jokes, but this joking scorn is often a mutual relationship, and the similarity between *fa'afafine* and trickster figures is something I am only now beginning to explore. A western visitor might comfortably respond to these apparently rambunctious queens as familiar transvestite homosexuals but would be wrong. *Fa'afafine* are, in an ironic and decentring sense, all male and all female, simultaneously.

Earlier anthropological accounts of *fa'afafine*, and therefore of Samoan gender identity, have been woeful efforts, telling us more about the epistemological shortcomings of anthropology as a colonial discourse than they do about Samoans. Mead, among her other sins, reduced gender variation in Samoa to a pathology. Charmed as she was by Samoans tolerance of the apparently mis-gendered, she obfuscated the subtlety of Samoan practices by dismissing gender and sexual variation as a disorder comparable to mental retardation and insanity. Later efforts, such as Shore [1981], refined Meads perspective somewhat, locating these third gendered Samoans in a complex model of sexual identity as interior state, but in doing so he simply repeated the Meadian pathology model, characterizing *fa'afafine* as failed males or imitation females, inherently male but disappointing simulations of something other, something not quite healthy. More recently, Mageo [1992, 1998] has attempted to locate the *fa'afafine* historically as evidence of cultural stress, echoing Garbers argument about transvestitism emerging out of distress in the categorical order of a society [Garber 1992]. This is a more promising approach not only because it sites *fa'afafine* as a real sex but also because it recognizes that sex and gender as enactments are ongoing and politically wilful practices. However, for Maggeo, whatever their cultural salience, *fa'afafine* remain denatured males, something deployed in the service of the other, more real, sexes.

What none of these "descriptions" address is the manner in which gender in Samoa is enacted out of intersubjectivity rather than from a base of interior precoding. We tend to assume there is an unavoidable "nature" to gender, distinction written into the species. Gender distinction is deployed as prior to social discourse, as prior to the inscription of the body. This fails to account for just what is being attended to when we inscribe sex and gender on acting bodies. Attention may be determined by difference or similarity but it need not be. The mode of attention, that is the pre-objective state of subjectivity [Csordas 1993], determines how distinction is cathected in the social field because mode of attention, among other things, determines the authoritative site at which order can be enacted and engaged through embodiment and within the embodied physical world. Where mode of attention focuses on the interior and therefore invisible aspects of things, which for Western cultures is a recent shift to the invisible interior of the body only occurring as recently the last 300 years, certain features of identity are fetishized as prior to meaning, as prejudgments which foreclose meaning. They take on the power of what Northrop Frye called resonances, which shape what can be attended to by rendering the invisible superlatively visible and supreme in its ordination of the world. However, mode of attention can also be located in the field of action rather than of actor. That is, where mode of attention derives operative meaning from action itself, the invisible is made meaningful rather than determining meaning. Mode of attention in Samoa is located in the field of action and not in interior states and so our conventions for recognizing gender are disrupted, inappropriate, too limited.

We also tend assume that gender is encompassed by the inherent and inviolable and timeless discourse of domination, that binaries are given in the species, binaries which are ranked in a mode of violent over-determination and domination. Morally and political powerful distinctions of perversion may be generated by the violence embedded in binary oppositions in our milieu such that, for us, gender is subsumed within the other discourse of domination, of control, of limitation. For Samoans, however, attention is ordered from a different point of view. For Samoans, attention derives from intersubjective connection, that is, from action in the social field itself. They rarely presume, pre-limit gender — few names mark gender, Samoan has no gender specific pronouns. Difference is generated from action rather than being imposed on action as a limiting frame. The problem with Gender, with a capital "G," is that it is a theory about everyone which, on close examination, applies to no one in particular. I have never met a woman or a man, although I have often heard complicated ideas about what these creatures might look like, should I happen upon one in a dark alley. This is especially true in trying to apply my own gendering and sexing lens to Samoa.

Fa'afafine are necessary to Samoan sociality precisely because they site the transgressive quality of gender and sex in everyday life. Gender and sex are performed as persistent transgressions rather than as "natural submissions," something which I suggest is a core aspect of Samoan identity as an ongoing and embodied process. Because gender is present in its exercise, emerging in action rather than residing in the individual as a fixed quality, it is not possible to say a Samoan has gender except when doing it. And this is not simply doing things with genitals, a common error that assumes that what genitals do is inherently salient to what genitals are. Rather, enacting gender and sex in Samoa always involves a masking of the body beneath, effectively discarding the flesh in order to have a flesh which is, at least for the moment, gendered and sexed. The body in Samoa is always expressed as a disguise.

Because of this, and the *fa'afafine* taught me this every important lesson, penises are not male and vaginas are not female. They are instruments for engendering action, where appropriate. They vanish from the body when they are not needed. Unlike our carefully circumscribed genital modesty, for Samoans genitals are part of their disguise when they are engendering their relations. They are superficial, and are only ever superficially central in engendered action. It is not only *fa'afafine* but men and women as well who express their gender as a series of facets, aspects invoked when appropriate and elided when irrelevant. Samoan gender is virtual, present only when performed. Male, female and *fa'afafine* exist as framing traces and like much else in Samoan sociality, is more often honoured in the breach than in the observance.

This is ideal, monosyllabic, a telegraphic picture of Samoan gender and especially a too narrow description of *fa'afafine*. Things change and there is something happening in Samoa, a new order of distinction insinuating itself into Samoan gender identity. There are few references to *fa'afafine* in the early missionary accounts. For one reason, perhaps, the ingrained gender switching was unrecognizable to the early missionaries. For another reason, I think that transvetitism as an aspect of *fa'afafine* engenderment is more recent, is a different order of code switching which has accompanied the intrusion of an emergent repressive biological gender absolutism. That is, *fa'afafine* does not mean looking like a woman but acting in the manner a woman is anticipated to act in a closely circumscribed range of contexts—and like a male in other contexts. Because these distinctions were only ever emergent, it is likely early visitors missed a great deal of what was going on. The looking like, an attention to body surfaces as a natural artefact being disguised rather than a process of disguising something more fundamental, is a more recent intervention in gender performance. That is, *fa'afafine* have become like drag queens and some have adopted the semiotics of American drag. However, these drag defined *fa'afafine* are distinguishable from other *fa'afafine* by Samoans themselves. There are the street *fa'afafine*, the business *fa'afafine*, the back village traditional *fa'afafine*, the homosexual men. Finer and finer distinctions are being drawn. Gender absolutism, the investing of the invisible with the power to foreclose meaning prior to meaning itself, has accompanied the repressive tendencies of Christianization and the invention of what many Samoans describe as modern sensibilities. But it is only emerging in Samoa. It is this contrast which makes the action based mode of attention and the transgressive practice of body narrative and discipline in Samoa so compelling.

This is because the *fa'afafine* mimics both male and female, not inverting them but transgressing them in an institutionalized subversive mimesis. Repressively sexed and gendered categorization did not emerge in Samoan for any reason, I suspect, other than there is no social-evolutionary or developmental reason for it to always emerge. Therefore, there is no real need for its absence to be explained, but a compelling need to explain the consequences of this absence, both historically and in terms of ongoing social change, especially in embodied praxis.

The breakdown in to male and female, those experientially discoherent, but enforced, bodies visualized into male and female, is de-resolved by the *fa'afafine*'s play which denounces male and female by being either, thus speaking the conundrum of gender, that classifications more often than not violate rather than order experience. *Fa'afafine* demonstrate gender and sex as choices, belying the naturalness of male and female by enacting a voluntary body.

The ambiguity of *fa'afafine* today, the often incoherent attitudes towards them, seems a function of the fragmenting of the earlier *fa'afafine* practice into bounded interiorized subjectivities. Where Gerber, in the 1970's, found Samoans unwilling, if not generally incapable, of commenting on the interior states of others, today ascription of non-voluntary interior conditions is becoming more common place.

In a cognitively modernising Samoa, the etiology of gender is becoming more formalized, more rigid, more natural, and so the *fa'afafine* begins to appear as outside that natural order, as against nature. As of yet, this is still quite vague and underdeveloped. There is a nascent and obscure discourse of hetero and homosexuality which is poorly formed and quite inarticulate, even though its primary source is the educated religious person. There is also a nascent and obscure discourse of natural and unnatural genders. As one man put it, "god made men and women and men and women made *fa'afafine*. I think god was right but we wanted more. We pay for these things."

This is emerging, a developing story. For now gender remains prototypes— male, female, *fa'afafine* are short hand for a web of stories, relationships, inversions and interpretations. We fail in our project to understand when we assume that the nature of distinction is given in a universal concept of difference. Difference is a network and not a characteristic and it is in the practice of difference and embodiment that we approach an understanding of the meanings and processes of gender and sex. While distinctions between prototypically defined classes is becoming increasingly important, the work of gender and sex, like the work of embodiment in general, remains, in Samoa, ground in the differences between individuals, differences enacted by individuals from a ground, ultimately, of constructed similarities.

A belief that gender and sex express the invisible, a display of the inner self, marked by sex, needs to be reconciled with the Samoan practice of wearing their sexed and engendered bodies as a an ongoing process of disguise. By eliding absolute distinctions, Samoan gender and sex do not render the invisible truth visible but create a contextual truth about which the body is not so much syntax as an intonation. The transgendered have always been a problem for conventional theories of gender. Where they are not completely ignored, they are pathologized into a bodiless state where their representations become misrepresentations, where their understandings are relegated to delusions. But perhaps the *fa'afafine*, and the drag queens and twangy boys of our own coffee shops and street corners, offer, in the breaches of their erstwhile biological code, a salutary and challenging lesson. It is the sexed and gendered body itself which is a fiction, masking neither innate similarity nor elaborate fundamental difference.

To decipher this, that culture is the wilful encoding of space and the deployment of invented bodies, that bodies are both beneath the skin and beyond it, is at the heart of this book. To accomplish this, a theory of embodiment needs to locate the body in the calculation of proper physical presence. It needs to recognize not only what the body means but the manner in which the body is rendered meaningful. It needs to determine the mode of attention which operates prior to discourse and makes objective discourse possible. And it needs to determine what is seen, what is knowable about the body deployed in social space. That is, what aspects or sites on the body, or in the body, are salient and visible and what aspects are elided, disguised, or unrecognizable. It needs to accommodate to the problem that sexed and engendered bodies are only selectively present, that no performance is perpetual. It needs to understand the complex of implications embedded in a comment a young Samoan woman made to me one day:

> We do not need women's liberation in Samoa. Not because men
> and women are equal. Because men and women are the same.

At the same time, without denying the richness of Samoan gendering captured in that simple assertion, it is also fair to suggest that what can be said about one putative sex can be said with equal confidence about the others as well. While there are intriguing differences at specific social sites in the ways gendered or sexed individuals behave or are treated, the key to understanding these differences is to see them in the larger context of a fundamental similarity which is at the core of Samoan embodiment. This may seem counterintuitive, given so many decades of feminist scholarship, but my point is a simple one — difference is not universal. It needs to be demonstrated. My argument in this text is that similarity overpowers difference in the enactment of Samoan gendered and sexed bodies.

There is also another issue I will not discuss, but for different reasons. I will stress the fluidity and changeableness of *fa'a Samoa* [the Samoan Way] throughout, because the substance of embodying practices in Samoa is always undergoing transformation. Television, migration to America and New Zealand, and the increasing influence of formal education, have each been major sources of influence and change [Holmes and Holmes 1992; Ochs 1988:189-210]. However, this is no different than inter-island influences between Samoa and its neighbours, in the period before European contact. There has always been a process of fertilization and influence from outside Samoa which has been an important aspect of how *fa'a Samoa* is practiced as an emergent order of propriety and tradition. To overemphasize modernization as a source of change runs the risk of creating a false dichotomy between authentic and introduced Samoan practices, which would belie the flexibility, and inherent adaptiveness, which have always been a part of these practices. I will not address either the source or direction of change, except where it is directly and explicitly relevant to the descriptive point I am making. Without denying the importance of such an analysis, I want to suggest that before we can discern where influences and changes have come from, we first need to discern the ground of practice on which these influences and changes are engaged.

To engage these two complex and contentious topics, in other than the briefest way, would entail a completely different book than the one I have written, especially given the two critically different objectives I will pursue in this text. One is ethnographic. In describing aspects of embodiment in Samoa, this text adds to a growing body of ethnography on Samoa which has been published in the last decade.[9] Chapters 2 through 5 can be read as a straightforward ethnography of aspects of the Samoan body, building on this growing body of new work. They form an ethnography in the sense in which Jackson compares ethnographic discourse to Polynesian string figures used to tell and illustrate stories, that is, "a game we play with words, the thread of an argument whose connection with reality is always oblique and tenuous, which crosses to and fro, interlacing description with interpretation, instruction with entertainment, but always ambiguously placed..." [1989:187]. As such, this text wobbles back and forth between generalized assertion and critical retreat, as a way of engaging the intricacies of the subject I am exploring without foreclosing the discussion. My dear friend Albert once told me, after listening to me complain for several minutes about my other Samoan informants appearing to change their minds about things between one conversation and the next, "that I was too much in love with facts and not enough in love with truth." It was not until several years later that I began to grasp just what Albert meant by truth, that it was and remains something flexible, changeable, deeply uncertain and reliable only for the moment in which it occurs. If the body is what we do with it, what we make of it, then I think Albert was warning me that the truth is what we need it to be, in the specific moments in which we need it.

However, the second critical objective of this text is, I feel, more important. I advance an argument here to the effect that the body needs to be more closely attended to in anthropological study because, in the daily enactments of the body, the web of culture is actualized. What the balance of this text endeavours to demonstrate are the sorts of issues and analyses which an ethnography of the body needs to explore. In this very critical sense, the Samoan bodies I will describe in the remainder of this text are illustrations of a method for looking at bodies, as much as they are an example of the practice of embodiment. The model of the thoughtful body this text proposes by example will require looking more closely at the evidence of what people are up to with their bodies, connecting these acts and practices to the wider issue of constituting culture. The chapters that follow will explore one way of approaching the task of describing the relationships between bodies and ideas about bodies, and the day to day activities through which they create and recreate each other, not only as these come to be played out in the process of making health, but equally importantly as they are played out, and played if you will, in everything from knowing where to put ones hands in public to experiencing the transformations of a rite of passage such as marriage or, in Samoa, the investiture of a chief. Taken together, this text is cumulative and exploratory, while at the same time, theoretically elusive. I am generating and applying a model, at one and the same time, as a way of naturalizing the study of the body as social process by avoiding, wherever possible, that descent into philosophical abstraction which alienates the living body from the equally vital practices of thinking about, through, and with it. The chapters which follow should be read as different vantage points from which to survey the same geography. Like the early map makers devising their charts, while never losing sight of the shore that guided them, in what follows I triangulate several features of a metaphorical geography of the Samoan body, in order to begin to devise a method for making that geography sensible.

I started with a story about how the possibility that an *aitu* would push me off my bicycle made me sweat and grow pensive as I pushed my bike across a bridge in the village in Samoa where I lived. That night the *aitu* left me alone. Or did it? That I remember that night, my skin retaining its own recollection of the tension across my shoulders, of the sweat that tickled the corners of my eyes as I tried to peer over the abutment into the dark water below, suggests that my own body, my own process of being and doing a body in the world now contains the presence, and the clear and present danger, of malicious Samoan spirits. My body has been transformed and made a different body than it was before that and the many other nights I spent learning to understand Samoan bodies, learning to see the differences and the commonalities in the body that I was doing and in those that were being done around me.

Chapter 3

Finding Samoa: Life, Living and Culture

Nothing is so aggravating as calmness.
>Oscar Wilde

So much of this I saw with the literary eye, or with the aid of literature. A stranger here, with the nerves of the stranger, and yet with the knowledge...I would find a special kind of past in what I saw.
>V.S. Naipaul—The Enigma of Arrival

One afternoon, while clearing my shelves, I checked the indices of 11 introductory level anthropology textbooks that I had accumulated. Samoa appeared in each of the 11 texts. The only comparable entry was the generic "Eskimo," which also appeared in all 11. It would seem that no other society has been as scrutinized and analyzed as Samoa. This, at least, is the appearance.

Much of Samoa's currency in anthropology, however, has been the result of the personality, and public role, played by Margaret Mead. It would not be unfair to suggest that while Samoa appears to be one of the most well known societies in the catalogue of human diversity which anthropology has compiled, what, in fact, is well known, are Margaret Mead's use of Samoa as a way of telling, mostly Americans, something about their own lives. The images of happy-go-lucky tropical islanders, and of anxiety free teenagers romping in the Pacific surf, are less about Samoa, than they are about America.

Perhaps in response to the over-formalizing effect of this "use" of Samoa as a moral tale, other work in Samoa has been remarkable for its consistency and rigour, and for its emphasis on the fluidity of Samoan culture. Shore [1977], for example, analyzes the connections between action, role, and context, in Samoan identity and personhood, arguing that for Samoans, identity is something drawn from the circumstances a Samoan finds himself or herself in. There are, he suggests, no fixed and rigid roles or identities in Samoa, only raw material in the form of skills and relationships between members, through which Samoans negotiate and renegotiate their sense of who they are in the world.

39

In his 1978 thesis, Keene analyzes the central role of surveillance and visibility in Samoan social control. He describes how all social action in Samoa is carried out in public, with the effect that structures of social control are underdeveloped. Systems of formal punishment, fixed rules of behaviour, and strictly applied sanctions derived from a standardized formula of propriety, are not components of Samoan social life, because the remarkable "visibility" of Samoan sociality makes abstract and depersonalized structures of social control unnecessary.

Two different studies of Samoan psychology [Maxwell 1969; Gerber 1975] have also stressed the importance of contextualization and fluidity in understanding Samoan personality and social life. Gerber explores the cultural meaning of, and socialization into, patterns of emotional experience and expression, arguing that Samoan emotion is tied to the immediate experience of roles derived from particular contexts throughout a person's life. The range of recognizable emotions, and the forms of their expression, are not finite and invariable. Rather, emotional life in Samoa is changeable and flexible, within a frame of restraint, which shifts as the social context shifts. Maxwell's study of Samoan temperament explores how Samoan extroversion and friendliness is a function of this flexibility, arguing that Samoan personality is being constantly renegotiated as Samoans move through different contexts and conditions in their lives.

Disagreements among Samoanists, except for the acrimony of Freeman's attack on Mead [Freeman 1983], have most often been about the implications of this fundamental fluidity for understanding life in Samoa. Mageo, for example, criticizes Shore's description of a fixed nature/culture dichotomy in Samoan ideology, arguing that the concepts *aga* [socially appropriate characteristics of a given person in a given context], and *loto* [qualities of behaviour which resist social conditioning], need to be understood as situational and interpenetrating, and not as essential and fixed qualities in Samoan self awareness [Mageo 1989]. Shore [1981], on the other hand, critiques the over-formalized model of gender Mead applies to Samoa. Instead, he argues, gender in Samoa is constituted in a flexible combination of gender and other social identities, sexuality and sexual desire, and reproductive responsibility, making gender roles changeable depending on the context in which they are performed [Shore 1981]. Schoeffel [1979] argues for a more critical understanding of the fundamental role the brother/sister dyad plays in Samoan social structure, a point taken in a different direction and to telling effect in Mageo's very recent analysis of gender and sexuality as the discursive fulcrum on which Samoan sociality and structural order, as well as Samoans capacity for adaptation and accommodation rests [Mageo 1998].

What each of these studies stress is that life in Samoa is never static. *Fa'a Samoa* (the Samoan Way) is a kind of short hand Samoans themselves use to indicate a wide range of things, from their perception of how their ancestors lived, to their persistent concern with propriety and a truly Samoan way of living, to the tension between what many see as the conflicting influences of tradition, and the need for modernization and development. *Fa'a*, as a prefix, is complicated because it indicates, among its other meanings, aspiration to something, that is, a causal path toward rather than a fixed code or standard. While *Fa'a Samoa* is spoken of as a totalizing code, it is a code which is sought after or pursued, rather than adhered to or obeyed. It is, as one informant put it to me, "a Samoan's dream of what Samoa should be," a process of desire, rather than a fixed standard of regulation.

This recognition has informed my own approach to Samoa, and the research reported and discussed in this text. The balance of this chapter describes the conditions of that research, and reviews, in general, the nature and structure of contemporary life in Samoa.

Methods and Intentions

This book is based on ongoing fieldwork conducted in Samoa, and in Samoan expatriate communities in New Zealand, Hawaii, and California since 1991, and is part of an continuing process on my part to understand what living as a Samoan means. My goal here is not to erect another elaborate anthropological model of Samoa but to offer a way of seeing Samoa which describes and articulates the intimate processes of everyday life. While in Samoa itself, I lived with a Samoan family, adopted as a "fictive" son and brother from the moment of my arrival, because of my friendship with the second oldest son, whom I had met while he was studying in Canada. Anonymity and confidentiality are important issues in fieldwork because, as anthropologists, we are often asking our informants to talk to us about things which are not only private, but may be secret or dangerous. Out of respect for my advisors and consultants in Samoa, and for their desire for confidentiality, all names, except those of my immediate family in Samoa, are pseudonyms. I use my immediate family's real names at their request. In all cases, I have discussed the issue of confidentiality with informants, and with my family, and have abided by each of their requests for privacy, not using information which was given to me in confidence, but not meant for public discussion. In the case of my immediate family, I discuss nothing in this text which violates the privacy of our homelife, always relying on information from other sources, even when the knowledge was so close at hand. To do otherwise would turn my participation in my Samoan family's life into an exercise in surreptitious observation rather than what it was, a relationship of affection and kindness. In some cases place names have been changed or omitted, although the name of the village in which I lived during my fieldwork, Vaimoso, has not been changed, at the explicit request of the villagers themselves.

As important, perhaps more important, this text is based on the determination I made to do whatever my hosts and hostesses did. I took as my starting point Michael Jackson's point about fieldwork and being a body, which I would like to quote in its entirety:

> Many of my most valued insights into Kuranko social life have followed from . . . [the] . . . cultivation and imitation of practical skills: hoeing on a farm, dancing, lighting a kerosene lantern properly, weaving a mat, consulting a diviner. To break the habit of using a linear communicational model for understanding bodily praxis, it is necessary to adopt a methodological strategy of joining in without ulterior motive and literally putting oneself in the place of another person: inhabiting their world. Participation thus becomes an end in itself rather than a means of gathering closely-observed data. . . . [T]o stand aside from the action, take up a point of view and ask endless questions, led only to a spurious understanding and increased the phenomenological problem of how I could know the experience of the other. By contrast, to participate bodily in everyday practical tasks was a creative technique which often helped me grasp the sense of an activity by using my body as others did. This technique also helped me break my habit of seeking truth at the level of disembodied concepts and decontextualized sayings. To recognize the embodiedness of our Being-in-the-world is to discover a common ground where self and other are one. For by using one's body in the same way as others in the same environment, one finds oneself informed by an understanding which may then be interpreted according to one's own custom or bent, yet which remains grounded in a field of practical activity and thereby remains consonant with the experience of those among whom one has lived. While words and concepts distinguish and divide, bodiliness unites and forms the grounds of an empathic, even universal, understanding. . . . The way learning to light a fire disclosed new understanding for me suggests that we might recognize a reality revealed through what we do which is at once the matter and the measure of what we say and think. After all, as the Kuranko adage says: "The word fire won't burn down a house" [1983:331].

Playing rugby or weeding gardens, helping care for young children, being treated by Samoan healers when I was sick, and receiving my own "Samoan" tattoo, are as important to this text as the formal interviews, questionnaires and surveys I employed during my fieldwork. Throughout my stay I performed the duties expected of a son, brother, and uncle and participated in all the daily work and concerns as a family member, responsibilities which I have maintained with varying success since my return to Canada by participating in important family decisions, and by contributing financially to family projects as an overseas son. I listened and watched and did as my family did, enveloping myself in the day to day labour and pleasure of life in Samoa as intimately and consistently as my status as a 'white, educated, older unmarried man' would allow. I combined formal data collection, the aggregation of things people say when directly questioned, with the personal experience of living and working as a member of a family, walking a line between participant and investigator which is not always easy to sustain, but which is at the heart of anthropology as a method of seeing the world. The resulting data, both in the formal sense of interview transcriptions and questionnaire coding data, and in the sense of the experience of living with, and as a part of, a Samoan family, which is inscribed in my memory and on my skin, combines practice and practicality in a web of different kinds of knowledge which, when taken together, serve as the foundation of a personal, but rigorous understanding.

With Jackson's insights in mind, this text is always as much about my own presence as an enacted body in the Samoan social field, as it is about the bodies of Samoans around me. A major irony is unavoidable: in writing about the body being done by Samoans, I am writing as a body engaged in its own enactment. My own embodying experience shapes and defines what I am seeing and doing as a body trying to light a fire in the rain while a group of Samoan boys watch and quietly laugh. Reflexivity begins and ends with this recognition on my part, that what I saw and did, and what I say and do now, are filtered through my own embodying practices — of coming to experience illness, both of those around me and my own, as Samoan experiences; of climbing coconut trees, tentatively, and with my eyes firmly trained on the ground below me; through the hours spent with the young men of one village clearing and re-clearing a cyclone-damaged taro garden; through the deaths of loved ones and friends, both while in Samoa and since; through the fights I narrowly escaped, and through the acts of intimacy and connection, and the acts of privacy and exclusion, that pervade everyday life. One thing that I firmly believe must be at the core of a model of embodiment is this sense that in studying bodies, our own callouses and machete cuts, illnesses and desires, are as important a part of the field research as the notebooks of myths and interview protocols that weighed down my suitcase on my return home [see also Rosaldo 1989:1-21].

The balance of this chapter is a general review of what can be reasonably asserted about the nature and mechanics of everyday Samoan life.

To do this, I combine previous work on Samoa: Shore's work on the political structure of Samoan society [1977, 1982], Mead's discussions of childrearing and social control [1961, 1969], and recent work by linguists [Ochs 1988; Duranti 1994] on the constitution of Samoan social order through language learning, and through speech acts. I have also been guided by Holmes's critical reproduction of Mead's earlier work [1957], and by his discussion of changes in Samoan village life, from the 1930's to the 1980's [Holmes 1958; Holmes and Holmes 1992]. To these sources I add my own data and interpretations, not so much building on their work as adding a different point of observation. By looking at *Fa'a Samoa* from the body up, I am expanding on the work of previous researchers, by taking their work in a new direction.

This combination of formal written sources with my own field experiences, necessarily produces an incomplete, mosaic-like, and very formal portrait. Any attempt to describe Samoa in a unitary and totalizing way cannot avoid the danger of over-directing interpretation and understanding, at the expense of both the diversity in Samoa, and of the ongoing, transgressive qualities of *Fa'a Samoa*. Milner, for example, comments on the "bewildering number of ways in which [common themes in Samoan culture] are worked out in villages" [1966:7]. There is, as Hovdhaugen [1987] and Love [1991] note with respect to Samoan "myths" and folktales, a wide range of variety between villages and districts in Samoa, not only in the form and content of stories told, but in their meanings and implications. This feature, of great variation in a geographically constrained society, makes general comments on what Samoans believe, or what Samoans think, difficult. In describing the basic features of contemporary village life within which Samoans live, I want to stress an important caveat. When I speak of Samoans, I am always speaking of the finite group of people with whom I lived. I was lucky because my adoptive Samoan family had strong and wideranging ties throughout the country, allowing me to work among diverse groups of people during my stay. While I do believe it possible to make very general assertions about certain fundamental aspects of *Fa'a Samoa*, I believe such assertions must always be framed more as possibilities than standards, as statistical probabilities rather than fixed, agreed-upon rules. What this review describes is a sense of the structure, light, and sound of daily life in Samoa.

To do this, I first need to lose sight of the body, and offer a kind of aerial view of Samoan's sense of their relationships to history and the modern world, before concluding with a sketch of the social geography of daily village life. Doing this defines the overall ground on which, and through which, Samoans deploy their bodies in their everyday engagements with culture and meaning. By exploring Samoans own sense of their mythical

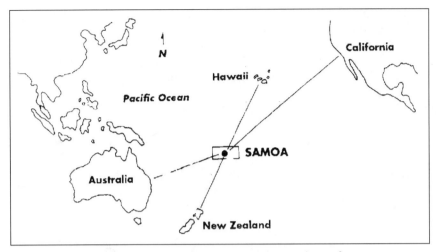

Figure 3.1 Location of Samoa in the South Pacific.

past, the current constellations of authority and conflict in politics, the family, and between generations, and the regular give and take of village life, I will provide the reader with a basic sense of the structures, practices, and concerns within which Samoan's live.

Between the Devil and the Deep Blue Sea: Samoans and Their Histories

"Samoa is an accident, I think?" Albert told me one afternoon.

Albert was somewhere older than 75, an untitled man who lived in an interior village several minutes by car from Apia, the capital of Samoa. When I first met him, he was sitting with friends drinking *'ava* [piper methysticum], a mild intoxicant used in many Pacific societies, at the large market in Apia. This ongoing circle began near dawn and could continue late into the night, mostly older men sitting and talking. I had passed them several times, carrying bundles of food to my family's pickup truck. Finally, he motioned me over and had me bend down so he could whisper in my ear.

" Are you one of those *palagi* who come here to marry our Samoan girls?"

I explained that no, I was a student living with a family in Vaimoso studying *Fa'a Samoa*. He laughed at this, and asked if he really was finally meeting Margaret Mead. Then he got the attention of his fellow drinkers and explained to them, in Samoan, who I was, a "very old schoolboy." The other men nodded or mumbled back at Albert who then beckoned me to let him whisper in my ear again. He told me to come and visit him whenever I wanted to find out the real truth. I didn't visit him for a number of months, and even then, only by accident. That accident turned out to be a turning point in my stay in Samoa, as Albert became a close friend and a sophisticated corrective to my lapses into misapprehension.

"An accident, Albert?" I asked. "One hundred and sixty thousand people bundled together on two tiny islands in the middle of the ocean is a big accident."

"One hundred and sixty thousand people bundled together on a couple of stones lost by God," he retorted with a cough. "And it is four tiny islands. You always forget Apolima and Manono. You are like all the other Samoans, there is only Upolu and Savai'i and then, always, America."

"But an accident, Albert. What can that mean?"

Samoa and the Dark Times [1]

Samoa was formed, according to one of the many origin stories I was told, in the darkness of the time before the coming of the missionaries, by the supreme god Tagaloa throwing several stones over his shoulder into the sea. They landed with a splash, and the long history of Samoa's journey into the light begins with the sun slowly filtering though the spray. It was a time of cannibalism, killing and war, famine, and invasion by neighbouring peoples, particularly by Tongans. The original union of the 35 islands in the Samoan archipelago was in a state of almost constant war, according to most Samoans today. These wars, the fires of which were the first sight missionary John Williams had of Samoa on his arrival in 1830, were most intense on the islands of Savai'i and Upolu, the largest islands in the archipelago, and the main islands of the modern Independent State of Samoa [Moyle 1984:69].

The environment of the Samoan archipelago is rich and tropical. The islands are volcanic in origin, with rich soil, and a pattern of rain-fed rivers and streams which make horticulture possible almost anywhere but in the central lava-plain of the largest island of Savai'i. Many of the islands are fringed by reefs whose waters are abundant with fish taken expertly by Samoan fisherman whose methods today have not changed notably from those described by the earliest missionary visitors [Stair n.d.; Barnes 1889; see also Buck 1971 (1930)]. Horticulture, mostly of tubers such as taro, and of breadfruit, coconut, and bananas, is the foundation of Samoan subsistence, a system of shared garden labour on land attached to *matai* [chiefly] titles, providing food for often very large extended families ['*āiga*]. Samoan horticulture is labour intensive though not extremely time consuming, aided by annual average rainfalls of between 5000 and 8000 mm, cooling winds ten months of the year, and reliable sources of clean water from mountain streams which cross most of the islands [Ward and Ashcroft 1998; Fox and Cumberland 1962].

"But why an accident, Albert?" I asked.

"God forgot Samoa, he left Samoans to fight and to kill each other and to waste their land and their food for hundreds of years. He left us somewhere in the darkness for hundreds of years and he almost forgot to come back."

"But God did come back, didn't he?" I asked, recalling the accounts early missionaries had published about their welcome in Samoa.

"John Williams told God that Samoans were still here in the darkness waiting for him to come back," he explained, smiling, and throwing several small stones over his shoulder at the pig that had fallen asleep behind the rock where we sat.

From 1830 onward a regular stream of missionaries, mostly from the London Missionary Society, came to Samoa, not because Samoa was in special need of Christianization, but because Samoa was among the easiest missionary exercises in all of the South Pacific [Gilson 1970:70-74]. Conversion was invited by the Samoans themselves, rather than inveigled by missionary persuasion or duplicity, because Samoans had been waiting for the arrival of the missionaries. The "goddess" Nafanua, who is variably described as the sister, cousin, wife, or aunt of the supreme god, Tagaloa, had predicted that sailing gods would arrive in Samoa from the east, bringing with them a special command from Tagaloa to improve *Fa'a Samoa* by acknowledging the sovereignty of these new gods as expressions of Tagaloa's will. Jesus came to Samoa and was welcomed like a returning son. The time of darkness, barbaric misconceptions, and brutal wars, ended with the return of God to his "forgotten" islands. Samoa, most modern day Samoans believe, has never been better than it has been since the arrival of God, moving out of the darkness of their isolation from the gods, forward into a time of light and prosperity and progress. Today the pre-European period is often referred to as the dark times, as Samoa's night, or as the time before Samoans could see.

This history, of a pagan horde labouring in the darkness until Christianity came to free them of their savagery, is a story told, with variation and embellishment, throughout the islands of Samoa. It is enshrined in the telling of *fagōgō*, "old stories" told at night as entertainments in the back villages, and on a weekly Samoan language radio program sponsored by the Methodist Church of Samoa. It is recalled in special versions of prayers which emphasize the biblical description of Jesus as the "way, the truth, and the light." It is reflected in the often critical, dismissive, or at least uncomfortable, attitude of many Samoans towards the myths and legends of old Samoa, collected now in illustrated volumes sold at the Methodist bookstore in Apia.

This version of the past, perhaps best described as the official version, is of central importance in Samoa because of the way it locates Samoans in the modern world, as a progressive and forward looking society that legitimately belongs, not as a newcomer, but as a longstanding participant in global history. It is a version of history Samoans use to distinguish themselves from what they see as their more barbaric island neighbours, and to establish themselves as peers in their dealings with the rest of the world, especially America. It is, however, not the only version of their history of importance to their everyday sense of being Samoan.

Politics and the History of the Fighting Brothers

The 35 island Samoan Archipelago is divided into three political units. American Samoa remains a semi-independent territory within the United States. Rose Atoll, a small coral island, is claimed by New Zealand. The remaining islands make up not only the largest land mass in the archipelago, but also the first independent state in the South Pacific. With Samoa's official independence from United Nations trusteeship in 1963, over 100 years of administration by Europeans, first Germany and then New Zealand, ended in the formation of a constitutional parliamentary government. This independence did not come without bloodshed and open revolt by Samoans.[2] In 1929, leaders of the Mau movement, an indigenous Samoan independence movement, marched on the offices of the New Zealand High Commissioner Apia. The police fired upon the crowd of Mau supporters, killing their leader, Tupua Tamasese, along with several others. In the ensuing years, the Mau continued to agitate among the leading *matai* [traditional chiefs] of the day, and a petition for independence was filed with the United Nations after World War II. Sixteen years of negotiations followed until a final form of constitutional rule was agreed upon.

The Mau were particularly active in the villages of Vaimoso and Pesega where I worked. During the cyclone in 1991, the bandshell in the centre of Vaimoso, which had served as the Mau headquarters, was destroyed, only its round concrete platform remaining. In the weeks, and then months, following the storm, debates sprang up among residents in the two villages over the question of restoring the bandshell, on which a weathered sign had once marked its role in the 60 years of agitation for independence. It was finally decided that, rather than the villages pooling their resources to rebuild the structure, the *matai* from all the surrounding villages should petition the government to restore it as a national shrine.

A controversy then developed over which *matai* should formulate the petition. It was argued that the Mau represented all of Samoa in their struggles and that, therefore, all *matai* should want to join in the petition to rebuild the bandshell. This was countered with the argument that the Mau was not a national movement, but a political party devoted to the furtherance of the aims of one of the two paramount "sacred chiefs" [*ali'i*] in Samoa, Tupua Tamasese. The *matai* for whom the other paramount *ali'i*, Malietoa, was their ultimate leader, insisted that they would not participate in the petition since the Mau had fought to exclude Malietoa from participation in the constitution as head of state. This was then countered by the Vaimoso matai with the argument that, since the constitution elevated both Malietoa and Tupua to the position of head of state, the old rivalry between the two titles was no longer relevant, the most important fact being that the Mau were instrumental in bringing the warring titled families together in a single Samoan government. Malietoa's supporters answered that the constitution had not brought the two families together because, while the current Malietoa had shared the title of head of state with Tupua at the time of independence, when this Malietoa died, the followers of Tupua would ensure that the new Malietoa would be excluded from the head of state position.

The situation I have just described typifies many of the political and social relationships in Samoa today. Samoan social order is built around relationships between title holding *matai*, who head their extended families ['*āiga*], and who stand as points of connection between all members of the '*āiga* and all other '*āiga*. This complex system of relationships is based on affinal kinship among members, and all Samoans can calculate their relative relatedness to almost any Samoan they happen to meet. Samoans distinguish between two forms of their extended family, the '*āiga*, which includes only those relatives who live in direct regular contact with each other in the same or related villages, and the '*āiga potopoto*, which is the entire congregation of related extended families. The '*āiga potopoto* are calculated by the relationships among *matai* contained in the *fa'alupega* or genealogies of *matai* [Charlot 1990; Kramer 1994]. However, these genealogies are undergoing constant revision and manipulation as new alliances, either through negotiation or marriage, create new kin relationships among matai. The '*āiga potopoto*, the broader group of connected small '*āiga*, is activated only in the event of some occurrence of an extraordinary nature such as the death of a paramount *matai*.[3] Throughout this text '*āiga* will refer to the smaller form of the extended family, the makeup of which is illustrated in Figure 3.2.

Any member of an '*āiga potopoto*, either male or female, can, potentially, become matai of their or any other extended family to which they are related, and move up through the system of ranked titles toward the highest status titles in the system. Shore [1982:80] distinguishes between rank and status in the *matai* system, where status is the fixed relationship

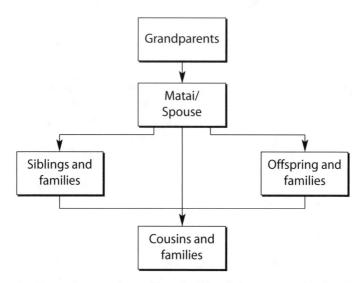

Figure 3.2 Members of *'āiga* by relationship to *matai* head.

of asymmetrical connection between *matai* titles encoded in the chiefly genealogies [*fa'alupega*], while rank is the real-historical relationship of deference and obedience between title holders [and their *'āiga*] which are a function of the current constellation of obligations and allegiances among title
holders. Status, in Shore's sense, orders the *matai* system, while rank drives it. However, Samoan's themselves actually use status as a strategy in
their dealings with members of other *'āiga*, as strategic, specific and circumstantial manipulation rather than a formal code of order. They are
expert at deploying the published versions of the *fa'alupega* as a tactic,
and as expert in generating their own contingent interpretations of these
texts as conditions require. In this text I will use the terms interchangeably to refer to the current relations of authority and allegiance between
title holders since in practice it is not possible to distinguish between the
ordering of status embedded in the *fa'alupega* and the exigencies of ranking that operate in the day to day negotiations and obligations between
matai and their *'āiga*.

All members of an *'āiga* are subject to the authority of their *matai*, and
each *matai* is subject to the authority of those *matai* ranked above them
in the hierarchy. Such a system is open to manipulation and conflict because the most successful *matai* are those who can use their knowledge
of kin relations across *'āiga*, to the advantage of their own extended family. The current system of chiefly ranking and authority continues today
in much the same way as it did at the time of the original missionary visits to Samoa in the 1830's [Gilson 1970:56-59]. Figure 3.3 illustrates the

structure of related statuses in this system. Competition both for access to these ranked titles, and competition between holders of these titles, is often fierce, as control of 80% of the useful land in Samoa is tied to these titles. Traditionally all land was attached to matai titles [and not to the title holders themselves, control of the land passing with the title to the successor]. Even with the alienation of some land to private or government ownership, subsistence in Samoa is still dependent on access to this customary land. While control of access to titles, which may be held by either men or women, depends to some extent on the good graces of the title directly above a given title in the ranking system, accession to titles is primarily controlled by members of the 'āiga, who meet to achieve a consensus on who should be granted titles over which they claim genealogical ownership.[4] Once "elected" by his or her extended family, a matai is expected to work on behalf of his or her 'āiga in relations with other families, in dealings between the various political districts, and in relations between families and villages and the central government. While normally held for life, chiefly titles can be taken away by the family if they become dissatisfied with the title holder's performance of his/her duties.

Competition and conflict across these different ranks is not over material resources. All land is alienated to the titles in perpetuity, and while enmity over the opening of new arable land may have been a problem deep in Samoa's past, today all possibly useful land is accounted for. Instead of material, matai compete for status capital, a kind of bank account of dignity, which provides direct material benefits for the members of the extended families led by their matai. Benefit is derived for the most part through the expansion of kinship relationships. All members of extended families are entitled to require assistance and support from any person with whom they have a measurable kin relationship. The wider the range of kin relationships a person can invoke, the better off they are. The extent, and the rank, of kin ties between 'āiga, as a result of marriage, determines the overall success and status of that 'āiga. Competition between matai, therefore, is for better, and higher ranking, kin ties, which enhances their account of status capital and allows them to attract or negotiate even better kin ties.

Competition takes the form of ceremonial exchanges of produce, pigs and ie toga [pandanus leaf mats], which take place at any important event involving more than one 'āiga, such as funerals, weddings, births, and the investiture of title holders. In these exchanges [fa'alavelave, literally, to make or do something complicated] matai from each participating 'āiga make cross presentations of goods, accumulating status capital by the wealth they are able to give away [cf Weiner 1992]. These exchanges can be massive in scale, drawing on the resources of all members of the 'āiga potopoto to provide the various goods for exchange and presentation.

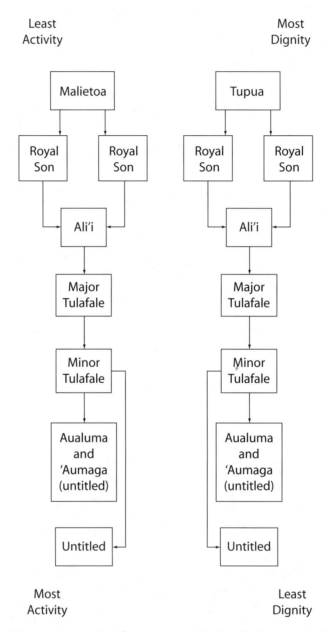

Figure 3.3 Samoan status classification system [idealized], showing the direction of increased dignity and of increased obligations of physical labour.

Matai making the presentations calculate the value they have to spare, the status capital which will accrue to them from the presentation, what status goods they will gain from the cross presentations which the receiving *'āiga* will provide them. In the weeks leading up to a *fa'alavelave*, the highest ranking *tulafale matai* of the *'āiga* involved will gather their resources, and calculate the size and components of the presentations they will make. They will calculate both the status wealth their presentations will earn them, and project these calculations into the future, taking account of *fa'alavelave* which they anticipate they will participate in the months ahead. At the same time, in drawing together their resources they will calculate every connection of obligation and duty they have formed with other *'āiga*, and call in those obligations, carefully measuring their material needs against the cost to them in status capital of releasing other *'āiga* from obligations to them. At the end of this, sometimes massive amounts of goods will be transferred, but it is important to note that the accumulation of these exchanged goods is not, at least primarily, for their material value for consumption. Rather, the goods received by an *'āiga* during a *fa'alavelave* are, for the most part, distributed among *'āiga* members in order to be stockpiled for use in future exchanges. Usually only perishable food items are consumed.

The competition at the heart of this system is rich and complex and would require more space and more detailed analysis to appreciate fully, because the *matai* system is at the heart of all Samoan social relations.[5] It institutionalizes a long standing relationship of competition and conflict in the system of political and social leadership. This antagonism is at the heart of contemporary national politics and informs political decisions and political controversies between *'āiga*, between villages and between political districts. It has resulted, quite recently, in the assassination of a government minister, and a parallel example of this in-built competitive structure can be seen in the coup, and its aftermath in Fiji in May 2000. It is the second version of Samoa's past encountered regularly in Samoa.

This competition is often characterized as an obstacle to Samoan development and progress and is the butt, even among high ranking *matai*, of great humour, and ironic commentary. Yet it remains the central defining feature of almost all Samoan social organization, determining where people may or may not live, where they can or cannot farm or travel, whom they vote for in national elections, and even which churches they attend. The *matai* system writes in daily political practice the long history of Samoan kinship and conflict, and sustains and re-writes that history deep into the future. It bridges ambivalence about the "dark times" with the practical exigencies of kinship, access to resources, and the need for some path to consensus and leadership.

Tattooing: History Written on the Skin

A final "use" of history is important for the way the body, through tattoos has become intimately implicated in the enactment of Samoan nationalism. Many anthropologists have written extensively about the invention of custom in the south Pacific and elsewhere [Keesing 1992, 1989; Borofsky 1987; Handler and Linnekin 1984; Linnekin and Poyer 1990; Hanson 1989; Hobsbawm and Ranger 1983; Wagner 1975], paying particular attention to how the deployment of revitalized tradition is an important part of emergent national and ethnic identity. That Samoan nationalism revitalizes tradition is not interesting because it is unusual, but because of the way the body is used as one of the primary sites for this historical renewal.

There are three key themes in Samoan tattooing: strength, endurance, and service [Franco 1991:134]. I want to reserve a detailed discussion of the implications of tattooing for an understanding of the Samoan body until later. Here I want to consider only the appropriation of tattooing, with its emphasis on strength and endurance, in the service of a new sense of nationalism. Historically, Samoan tattooing of men marked, among other things, servitude. Untitled men received extensive body tattoos in their early twenties, tattoos which then signified their role of server to *matai*. This is a key relationship in Samoa, referred to as *soa*. The *soa* relationship is a kind of mid-state between different positionalities, in this instance between the *matai* and those over whom he has authority. The relationship between *ali'i* and *tulafale* is also a *soa* relationship, the *tulafale* acting as a go-between, if you will, between the two rankings of chief. *Soa* relationships have other, more intimate, manifestations, including a friend who acts as interlocutor in courtship, and, as well, the relationship of support and assistance between adolescent boys, a specific relationship I will return to in a later chapter. Body tattoos indicated the young man's willingness to follow his *matai* and to subsume his own aspirations in the service of the needs of his *matai*, a position of obligation, submission, and service Samoans refer to as *tautua* [Mageo 1998:55].[6] Later in life, these tattooed men were rewarded with titles of their own in recognition of their service, which suggests we read the traditional tattoo as incorporating service, self-effacement and humility in the over-all process of acquiring authority in Samoa [McGrevy 1973].[7] Indeed, in the pre-European period, "tattooing was necessary for a chief to hold his title and an untattooed chief was unheard of" [Forsyth 1983:58].

Missionaries zealously stamped out the practice of tattooing, mostly because the loyalty to *matai* was thought to interfere with loyalty to the pastor and thus to God. It has been estimated that the practice of traditional tattooing was completely eliminated within 30 years of the arrival of the first missionaries [Forsyth 1983]. Missionaries, successful in almost totally converting Samoans to Christianity, exercised a great deal of effort eliminating Samoan body practices. The first to go were the night dances [po'ula] which were often mounted as village entertainments for travelling parties of matai [malaga] engaged in political negotiations. These were banned because they often had carnal finales carried out in the bush surrounding the village. The missionaries then banned traditional hairstyles [involving shaving the head of everything except a long pony tail] and finally, traditional body tattooing. This focus on reshaping the surface of the body, as a measure of the reshaping of the soul is characteristic of Christianity's division between the carnal and the spiritual body [Greenberg 1988; Foucault 1980]. It recognizes that what is expressed on the surface is not separable from what is being thought inside and that re-forming one is necessary to reform the other. Inside and outside are the single frame of the sacred, something which Samoans understood readily because it is a key aspect of their own sense of morality and embodiment.

Tattooing was renewed during the most active period of Mau agitation for independence in the 1920's and 1930's, but its renaissance was much more extensive in the years immediately following independence in 1963. Tattooing in several forms is now widespread throughout Samoa. Of interest here are the tattoos both men and women are receiving as markers of their status as "true" Samoans. Some of these are traditional in form, such as the taulima, a bracelet like tattoo on the wrist which, in the past, was reserved for the sons of high ranking matai. Others are borrowed from throughout the Pacific, particularly from Maori patterns. Finally, others are classic "biker" tattoos of dragons and busty women.

This apparently indiscriminate tattooing was originally something only the roughest of men, specifically town taxi drivers, were noted for. Any village youth getting a tattoo of this sort was the object of either humour or criticism for taking "taxi drivers" as role models. However, in the last several years this practice of decorative tattooing has become more and more widespread. What may, originally, have been tied to issues of masculinity, and to the rough and ready subculture of the taxi driver, has now spread to women, school boys, Samoan professionals, and even some younger matai.

The most common explanation offered my questions about tattoos among younger Samoans was that it "showed everyone I was strong like a real Samoan should be." Many people were explicit that part of their desire for a tattoo derives from the fact that it had been banned by the early missionaries and European governing bodies, because something of the traditional Samoan values of strength and the ability to endure pain had been taken away from them by these early, somewhat punitive, re-strictions. There is a widespread sense among many younger Samoans that the modern world is taking away many of the better features of Fa'a Samoa, particularly those of courage and fortitude, generosity and service, and respect for tradition. While it is acknowledged that many of these tattoo figures are not traditional in design, the key issue for Samoans is the act of getting the tattoo, rather than the specific symbols etched into the skin. Having a tattoo has become, for many younger Samoans in particular, a symbol in itself, a symbol of their Samoanness. However, this symbolism was not solely the reasoning of younger Samoans. In the weeks following Cyclone Val in 1991, my adoptive family, including my *matai* father, suggested I receive a tattoo, a *taulima*, to mark my own Samoanness as someone who had participated in the communal efforts during the storm. The new tattoo is, at least for many, an attempt to reclaim values and traditions of pre-European *Fa'a Samoa*, this time in the name of a Samoan ethnicity which marks being Samoan as a distinctive identity which transcends kinship, *'āiga* and *matai* ties. The *Fa'a Samoa* these younger Samoans are championing is grounded in a leveling of obligations of service, a drawing down of *matai* in order to connect their authority more closely with the *'āiga* itself, and a resistance to what many see as a global homogenization which, in their eyes, undermines the distinctive commitment to dignity, service, and physical and moral strength which is at the heart of their revitalization of *Fa'a Samoa* as a national identity. That is, the tattoo marks on the body a sense of national self-hood which attempts to reassert what many younger people see as the lost values of *Fa'a Samoa* as their ancestors practiced it. The politics of these assertions is intricate, combining the effects of the homogenizing influences of contact with other societies with the effects of Western style education, which has elevated a kind of abstract Samoan traditionalism as an object of formal reverence and study. What tattooing also appears to write into the skin is the development of a canonical form of *Fa'a Samoa* which opposes the relative powerlessness of the young against the failure of the old and powerful to keep to the truth of what these young people see as the "real" *Fa'a Samoa*.

The question of revitalizing authentic traditions relates less to the truth of the past than it does to the issue of who has the authority and power to authenticate [Bruner 1994], and points up a tension between the empowered elders and the powerless young in Samoan politics and ideology. Contemporary tattooing reasserts the story of how the original Malietoa, having taken up cannibalism as a true Samoan practice, was tricked by his son, who offered himself in disguise as a meal for his father. This disguise helped Malietoa learn the danger of his error, and return to a truer *Fa'a Samoa*. While issues of masculinity, of sex and sexual prowess, and even of class, are also embedded in the post-independence practice of tattooing, it is this "real Samoan history" explanation which is the most important to Samoans. It is another version of Samoan history, one which is inscribed, literally, on the skin. The renewed tradition of tattooing, if not

of traditional tattoos, marks the current generation of Samoans as standing in a contentious relationship to their own sense of their history, both
of the past and of their projected sense of their future, a contentiousness
which they are expressing with their skin.

There are other ways Samoans relate to their history. The one I find
most interesting is the "negrification" of Samoans by Samoans themselves,
which has its roots in the treatment some Samoans have experienced living in the large Samoan communities in Southern California. Many
Samoans, particularly younger men in American Samoa, identify with
African-Americans, and have adopted African-American slang, fashion,
and music. This is less prevalent in Samoa, where the major Black icon is
Bob Marley. However, among younger Samoans, especially males in high-
school, African-American fashion, and a sense of standing in relation to
"whites" in a way similar to African-American youth is gaining importance. However, I have chosen these three—the relationship between modern Samoa and the Dark Times before Christianity, the playing out in the
contemporary *matai* system of the longstanding historical antagonism between the two paramount chiefs of Samoa, and the strain between chiefs
and adults, and Samoan youth over who should control the definition and
revitalization of Samoan tradition—because they highlight the tension
that pervades *Fa'a Samoa*, a tension between being modern while retaining a sense of traditionalism. Whether it is a denial of the value of "old
Samoa," while retaining "Samoan traditions" in their Christianity, a sense
that the *matai* system is both necessary to Samoa's future, and a failure
because it is unable to overcome the longstanding tensions built into the relationships between *matai*, and among the *'āiga* they lead, or the revitalization of a Samoan identity based on strength and service, contemporary
Samoa is a contentious space in which values and ideals are tested, constantly reassessed, disposed of and reinvented. It is within this landscape
of histories that daily life, in its samenesses and varieties, is carried out.

The Town and the Tua: Daily
Life in Samoan Villages

Samoa comprises 11 volcanic islands, of which four are inhabited, with
a total landmass of approximately 2860 square km [Fox and Cumberland
1962:114] and lies 4300 km south-west of Hawai'i. Overall population
density is around 140 per square mile, based on the most recent census
data which gives the population at approximately 160,000 and 200,000
[per.comm, Samoan Department of Statistics]. However, this figure belies
the fact that village population density is considerably higher. Vaimoso,

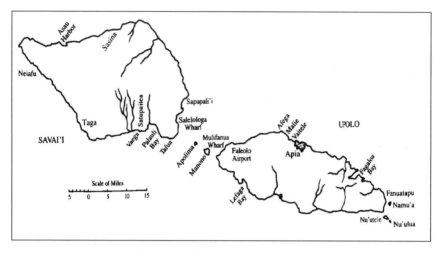

Figure 3.4 The Islands of Samoa

for example, has a density of 750 per square mile, because of the close concentration of households in the core of the village. The main islands of Upolu, where the capital area of Apia is located, and Savai'i, the larger, but least populated, are divided by volcanic ridges which form deep valleys running to the coasts. Upolu is now ringed by a single coast road which joins all areas of the island except the Aleipata district on the southeast coast, an area noted for both the excellence of its reef fishing and for its relative inaccessibility, surrounded as it is by high mountains and twisting passes. Along with the coast road, two main cross island roads link the north and south coasts. Savai'i is also ringed by a coast road which reaches all but the remote north-east corner of the island. Like Upolu, all areas of Savai'i are accessible, with varying degrees of difficulty, via several cross island and interior roads, including roads engineered and graded by villagers themselves.

Most villages are located along the coast road on Upolu, having moved from interior locations in the period following European contact [Gilson 1970]. Interior villages on Upolu are most often important agricultural centres, located in the midst of extensive village and government plantation lands. On Savai'i, villages cluster on the small coastal plain that rings the two major lava fields which form the centre of the island. The small islands of Apolima and Manono, located in the rough, windy strait between Upolu and Savai'i, are occupied by very small communities which, with devastating erosion caused by an increase in tropical storms in the last 30 years, are now dependent on linked communities on Upolu and Savai'i for food and supplies.

Almost all Samoans are engaged in some form of subsistence farming, growing taro, breadfruit, bananas, and coconut. All Samoan families keep pigs, the excess used for food, but which are reared primarily for presentation at ceremonial exchanges [fa'alavelave]. Away from the Apia town area, most villages will include several families who fish on a daily basis, fish being an important complement in Samoan's diet. Subsistence practices, while still producing almost half the staples of some family's needs, are no longer the sole source of food in Samoan villages. Quite often, especially in villages on the southern coast of Upolu, food is grown in small, family plantation plots adjacent to households, or in larger garden plots some distance inland from the village, primarily for use in fa'alavelave exchanges, and for the feeding of pigs. In villages further from the Apia town area, even villages with extensive garden holdings, food from gardens supplements their diet, the bulk of the produce being grown either for sale at the Apia market or for use in fa'alavelave. Ready access to town shops, and the presence of small shops in almost every village on the two main islands, provides the new Samoan diet with its basic components of frozen lamb parts, rice, and prepackaged noodle soups. While daily meals almost always include such basic ingredients as taro and boiled banana, it is now not unusual for families to reserve their own hand-grown produce for fa'alavelave and provide for their daily needs with market or shop purchases, even of produce they themselves grow in some abundance.

Samoa can be divided into two general forms of village, the villages of the Apia town area and the tua, or back villages. This distinction is one Samoans draw themselves. Town area villagers think of back village dwellers as simple, less developed, and less forward thinking, and back villagers treat town dwellers as poor examples of Samoan values and beliefs. However, in practical terms, day to day life is not very different between the two types of village, since access to town facilities, and the influences and opportunities of the developing cash economy, are equally distributed throughout the islands. Everyone lives in a traditional village, although people throughout the island often dispute the calibre and authenticity of "tradition" across villages, usually holding up their own living arrangements as more exemplary of Fa'a Samoa than those of even closely related villages.

This understanding followed months of confusion and misunderstanding that preceded my grasp of what the articulation of roads and open spaces and plantations meant in the villages I lived in. At first they all seemed a ramshackle and haphazard juxtaposition of concrete houses, traditional, open-walled fale, and tumbling down shacks, with roads and paths running akimbo from the main road traversing or circling every village. Months after my arrival, "when the land had more meaning, when it had absorbed more of my life" [Naipaul 1987:5] I came to understand and to feel that all Samoan villages have the same conceptual plan, although the physical layout of villages can be dramatically different.

Traditional villages are centred on an open green area [*malae*] around which are ranged the household compounds of the various '*āiga* who make up the village. The largest house in the village is usually that of the ranking *ali'i* chief. Behind this circle of residences is a second circle of buildings, including the cook house, sleeping quarters for younger family members, and an area for feeding and caring for the family pigs. Beyond this lay a ring where the toilet houses [*fale vao*, literally, forest houses] are located, near the plantation land. Beyond this lies the bush, undeveloped, but still owned, green space between villages. As I will explore more closely in Chapter 7, when I discuss Samoan anatomy, there is a distinctive and direct relationship between village layout, the functions of each part of the village structure, and Samoan embodiment, the village and the individual body standing in a homologous relationship such that each resembles the other.

With population expansion, especially in the decade following the influenza epidemic of 1918, and accelerating sharply in the mid-1940's [Harbison 1986:68-69], and with the slow movement of more and more people into what would become the villages of the town area, villages along the southern coast of Upolu, and in the area of the government harbour and wharf on Savai'i, began to lose their roughly circular form as the living areas encroached on both the *malae* and the immediately contiguous plantation area. The effect of this was the emergence of more closely circumscribed '*āiga* compounds within villages, and the pushing of village plantation land further and further away from the village itself. While villages conforming to the older pattern of circular distribution are still common in the areas further from the Apia town area, the general influence of a steadily increasing population has led almost all villages to at least begin to abandon their open form.

The village of Vaimoso, where I lived and worked during my stay in Samoa, is located in the heart of the Apia town area, and this transformation from circular to less orderly village layout can be illustrated schematically. In Vaimoso in 1930 the central living area of the village, the malae, was still relatively intact in spite of the passage of the coast road, almost directly through the middle of the village. By 1991, when I was first living there, Vaimoso had been completely transformed by population expansion. While the *malae* remained, even with the wider and now paved coast road running through it, the conceptual heart of the village, living spaces had become fragmented, and isolated, within the finite village space. Plantation land had been overtaken by housing demands, and what plantations remained in the village were household garden plots, not unlike North American kitchen gardens, providing some basic foodstuffs for either daily consumption or for formal exchanges.

However, even with these changes, villages retain their traditional conceptual geography, an often explicit and clearly articulated public discourse of village social space, in which the village is divided into front and back, and into centre and periphery. The front/back distinction relates mostly to the kinds of activities which occur in each part of the village. The back end of the village is the space of manual labour, dirt, and detritus. The front end of the village is the area of politics and religion, of formal events, such as weddings, funerals and village meetings, and of socializing and play. In a sense, the front of the village is the place where one is a member of the community, while the back of the village is the place where one pursues more individualized activities. This front-back distinction applies at the household level, too, with the main *fale* in which all important family activities took place, making up the front of the household plot. The back buildings, that is the cookhouse and sleeping houses for younger family members, chicken coops and, finally, the toilet house, occupy the less visible and less social part of the compound. Finally, this front back distinction also applies to space within the main *fale* itself. These circular houses are divided into a front and a back space. The front space, marked by the front entrance, is the space where family socializing takes place, while the back space, marked by a rear entrance, is the less formal private space. This distinction operates not only in the kinds of activities that take place, but in how people outside the house behave in relation to the house. A visitor coming to the front of the house is required to either remove his or her shoes and enter the house or, at least, to seat themselves on the steps leading into the house, before engaging in conversation with someone in the *fale*. Someone approaching the house at the rear door is allowed to stand, either at the bottom of the stairs or in the entrance itself, and carry on their conversation.

The centre/periphery distinction refers to the relative dignity of the space and the activities which occur there, connecting the dignity of spaces to the level of social interaction and the degree of visibility. The centre of the village, focused on the *malae* and on the house of the most important *ali'i*, is the heart of the village, and the space of greatest social importance. It was and remains the space of greatest dignity. Dignity [*mamalu*] is a key concept in *Fa'a Samoa* and expresses, as one man told me, the "need to give away our own needs so that the needs of the *'āiga* are better served." One of Shore's informants put it even more clearly when he said that "if we lived according to our own desires, there would be no dignity in our culture. Things are kept well ordered in order to keep the culture dignified" [1981:163]. The dignified centre of the village is the core space where sociality and community are expressed and enacted. As one moves out away from this centre, and finally to the bush area around the village, the level of dignity decreases, until, in the bush, all sociality and communal attachment appear to evaporate.[8] Figure 3.5 illustrates this decrease in dignity the further one moves from the centre of the village. This pattern of

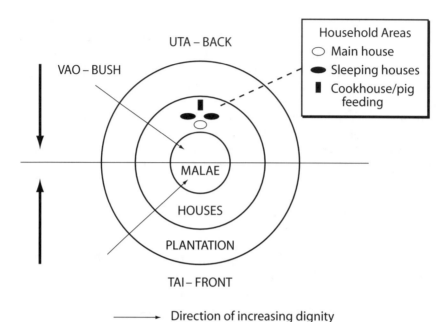

Figure 3.5 Concentric Circles of Dignity in
Samoan Social Space [after Shore 1982:68]

decreasing dignity is fundamental to Samoan's understanding of *Fa'a Samoa*.

What is diminishing as one moves away from the centre of the village is sociality itself, and in particular, surveillance [Shore 1982:67ff; Keene 1978]. The original circular village layout, combined with the open walled houses which one still finds throughout Samoa, formed the basic landscape of visibility by which all members of Samoan society were monitored and disciplined. Social life, for Samoans, is the life they see, understanding and seeing something expressed in the same word, *malamalama*. Appropriate and good behaviour [*aga*], is that behaviour which can and should be seen. As one moves away from this visible centre, it becomes increasingly possible to do things without being seen and, for Samoans, that which is done in secret, either intentionally or simply as a function of distance from the centre, is *lēaga*—asocial and dangerous [Mageo 1989].

Lēaga is a difficult concept to translate into English, even though its more mundane component, "bad," is most often given as its root translation. However, like all moral or ethical judgements, bad for Samoans embeds a combination of values and judgements which the simple word "bad" cannot adequately encompass. Bad, for Samoans, is that which is either directly anti-social, as in murder or theft, or that which is asocial, that is, things done in secrecy. However, along with these two senses, *lēaga* can also mean failing to meet your social responsibilities. As one man put it too me one day, "hitting your child when he is cheeky is good, is the thing you must do, and not hitting your child to teach him not to be cheeky, that is *lēaga*." So, unlike the English word "bad," which can be used to refer to everything from spoiled food to murder, *lēaga* directly implicates only those things which are specifically social and communal.[9]

This conceptual landscape of good and "bad" space, then, is preserved even in those villages which have completely abandoned a centre/periphery layout, so that even in rectangular village layouts with *'āiga* compounds butting up against each other or overlapping, it is possible to map the "rings" of decreasing dignity from the heart of the village [today either the meeting house of the most powerful *'āiga*, the home of the ranking *ali'i matai*, or the church which the most important *matai* attends]. If we look at Figure 3.6, which represents Vaimoso as it existed in 1991, we find that the two major distinctions of front and back and centre/periphery are still in force. The coast road which divides the village land serves as an approximate marker of the front and back of the village, the front being the area north from the tarred road, and encompassing the *malae*, and the households of the important *matai* attached to the ranking *ali'i* of the village. The centre/periphery marking of the village space is tripartite. The circle labelled 1, which includes the *malae* and the home of the ranking *ali'i*, indicated by the shaded circle, is the dignified core of the village of Vaimoso. Within this core all the households of important *matai* are to be found, along with the Methodist church, which is the church of the paramount *tulafale matai* of the village. Circle 2, encompassing the core, is the area occupied by *matai*, and their *'āiga*, who rank somewhat lower than those in the core. The final roughly defined ring, labelled 3, is the space of the lowest ranking families of the village, along with the few commercial enterprises found in Vaimoso.

Not illustrated here, but of equal importance to the overall marking of the village space in terms of dignity, each area within the village can be mapped by decreasing dignity such that in area 1, the most dignified and formally important area of the circle is that area immediately surrounding the home of the *ali'i*, the *malae*, and the home of the highest ranking *tulafale* attached to this *ali'i*. Similar mappings can be done around the households of highest ranked persons in each of the other two areas. The key events of village life, some of which I discuss in later chapters, such as *fono* [meetings of *matai*], village entertainments, and even village trials, all occur in the centre of circle one, while key events of importance to smaller groups within the village areas take place in the most visible and open area of the section of the village in which they live. I should note

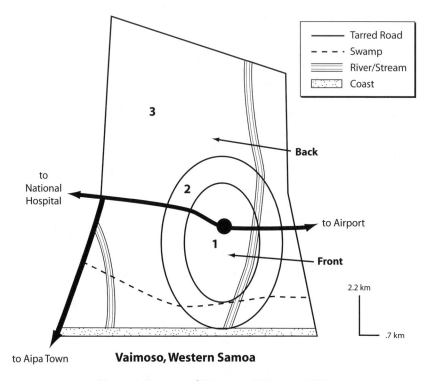

Figure 3.6 Areas of Dignity in Vaimoso, 1991

here, briefly, that these demarcations are not just abstractions which refer to ideas about propriety and sanctity. They have real consequences. Boys from circle one, the area of the village where my Samoan family resided, would often pick fights with groups of boys living in other sections of the village, and then retreat quickly into the area centred around the *malae* in area one, explaining to me that their antagonists would not follow and fight them there, because fighting in this area of the village would be "too *lēaga*."

This model of dignity and its relationship to visibility is expressed in other ways as well, for example, in distinctions between the inside and outside of houses and even within the household space itself. Traditional Samoan houses [*fale*] were unwalled platforms surmounted by steep thatched roofs on columns made of single logs. Gradually during this century, and with increasing rapidity since independence in 1963, these *fale* have been replaced by European style bungalows with small windows and tin roofs. The house has increasingly become a private space and the household unit, often including parents, children, one or more cousins or grandchildren and occasionally aunts and uncles, has increasingly become a private social unit. At the same time, however, markers of adherence to the tradition of visibility have developed, the most impressive of which are the large traditional *fale* of the ranking *matai* of the village. In many villages the ranking *matai*, usually the highest status *ali'i*, will live in a thatch roofed *fale* of monumental size, a fact people often explained to me as how they seek to preserve the integrity of their adherence to *Fa'a Samoa*. Within the private bungalows themselves, the "simulation" of the visibility of life in the *fale* is sustained with the building of large living areas in the front parts of houses which are often walled with un-draped windows, in a glassed-in impersonation of the wall-less traditional *fale*.

Another, more subtle way that visibility is maintained as the key of the sociality of the core of the village is in the layout of village roads and pathways. While more and more families have come to live in relatively isolating household compounds, compounds no longer ringed around a communal open area, village common paths and roadways are often laid out in such a way that they pass directly before the windows or doors of houses even though more easily graded routes are available. This placement of roads, and in some cases a proliferation of paths in and around even very small villages, is explained by many Samoans as being needed so that "we can see where people are going and what people are doing." The roads and paths at the heart of the village, along which village daily interaction takes place, have, in some instances, replaced the *malae* as the most dignified space in the village.

For example, in Vaimoso the most dignified area in the entire village is often not the *malae*, but the roadway directly in front of my Samoan father's European style house because Sei'a, my father, was not only the most important *tulafale* attached to the *ali'i* who was paramount in Vaimoso, he was also the ranking *tulafale* for the political district of which Vaimoso was the centre. His presence in some official capacity transformed this often very busy roadway into a space of great sanctity, a fact he was well aware of, when, prior to the start of a wedding party in our house, he took me out onto the roadway, commenting that "now I am going to make your little road into a church."

Finally, while the *matai* of most villages had control of land far in excess of the land needed for plantations, village expansion has tended to use every available metre of living space in the core of the village before expanding living areas deeper into the plantation or bush areas. In back villages where this process of change in village form is still continuing, it is not unusual to see houses being built such that they almost touch each other, while land outside the dignified centre of the village lies empty and unused, even for plantations. Samoans deploy their social existence in a space circumscribed by a concern for dignity and visibility and continue to maintain this centre/periphery distinction at the heart of even the most modernizing of efforts to transform the physical attributes of village life. It is a mapping of dignity which extends even to the way people talk.

There are two speech registers in Samoan. Formal or "good" speech, characterized by the presence of the consonant "t," is defined by Samoans as the appropriate speech register to adopt when speaking with someone of higher status than oneself, when speaking of matters of great importance, or when talking about private and personal things governed by a concern for modesty or propriety. So called "bad" speech, characterized by the replacement of most "t" sounds with the consonant "k," and by subtle, but inconsistent, changes in grammar, is the speech of everyday life. It is the speech of parents addressing their children, of equals conversing in private and so on. In one sense, at least, "k" speech is the register of friends and "t" speech the register of strangers. "T" spellings of words are also required in written Samoan.[10] As well as changes in pronunciation, there are also two vocabularies of common words, one for use in "good" speech and the other for "bad," informal speech. I will, throughout the chapters below, refer to conversations or words in terms of their being parts of either polite, "good" speech or informal, "bad speech," because at times using polite or the informal turns of phrase is important to the meaning the speaker is trying to convey. To give a mundane example, while it is possible to informalize person's names, such as transforming Matau into Makau, in doing so the speaker may be stressing the status difference between him or herself and Matau, expressing anger or disappointment with Matau, or be attempting to infantalize him. The use of the "k" in Matau's name can embed considerable information about the context of the speech and the intention and status of the speaker.

From village planning to the geography of appropriate kinds of space and activity to the manners in which people speak, the conceptual form of daily life is built on the pursuit and preservation of order, surveillance, and propriety.

A Day in the Life of a Samoan Village

Samoans are Polynesian people with light brown skin and straight dark hair. They are generally tall, about 6 foot, and, as they grow older, usually approach or exceed 200 lbs. They move throughout the villages in which they live with a slow, swaying gait. While younger Samoans have adopted fashions from overseas, in particular America, almost all Samoans wear the traditional Pacific wraparound skirt, known as a *lavalava* in Samoan. This skirt, and a t-shirt, are the most common outfit in everyday life in Samoa. These are a stately and robust people, physically. They take great pride in beautifying themselves, and even greater pride in their strength. While young men are usually well muscled and strong, young women are rounded, supple and sturdy. Mature men and women, on the other hand, are both massive, and each capable of comparable acts of strength and endurance. One very common career for Samoan men overseas is in professional football or in wrestling. Recently a Samoan was awarded one of the highest accolades in Japanese Sumo. It is difficult to describe Samoans physically except in terms of superlatives of size and, I hope to show, grace.

If the earliest missionary accounts are reliable, daily life in the villages of Samoa has, in general at least, not changed significantly in the one hundred and fifty years since the beginning of intensive European contact. The day begins around sunrise, when the young men of the village wake to feed the pigs and prepare the morning tea. Some of these young men will, after a shower and some hot tea, go off to the plantations directly adjacent to the village, or to plantation land further inland, to weed, plant and harvest crops as the season demands. Other young women and men will perform duties around their household compound, before preparing to go into town, or to one of the small manufacturing plants, government offices, or town shops, should they be lucky enough to have a cash job.

While the young men prepare the small morning meal, usually of tea and biscuits, older men (including *matai*) rise and spend some time cleaning and grooming the village common areas. Older women spend most of this early part of the morning supervising younger men and women in their chores, getting the older children ready for school, or visiting each other to plan the days activities. All villages on both Upolu and Savai'i are within easy walking distance of elementary schools, although not all children attend school.

Once the children, who have been dressed in their uniforms, are sent off to school and the young men and women have gone to the plantations or to their cash jobs, the older men and *matai* spend most of their mornings meeting with each other to talk about village affairs and to plan construction projects or village cleanups. Deference typifies these conversations and plans, regardless of the relative status of the participants. *Matai* and untitled men will spend mornings in these informal conferences, discussing and listening to each other's ideas and concerns before arriving at a consensus. While the paramount *matai* can and do sway the direction of village decisions, in some cases even controlling every aspect of village decision making, they do so according to strict rules of consensus and humility. In talking to people about their villages and their leaders, the English word most often used to describe good *matai* is humble [*fa'amaulalo*]. People explain that a good *matai* provides well for his *'āiga* in ceremonial exchanges and sustains the status and authority of his *'āiga* in relations between families and villages, but, at the same time, a good *matai* does not "show off," does not wield his power obviously and blatantly. A humble man, they explain, is a man who listens to other's concerns and interests, and always, at least explicitly, sets aside his own personal opinions, so that everyone in the circle of those concerned has a voice and a say. *Matai* are often criticized for being to bold and arrogant, and not enough like fathers. It takes humility, a young *matai* explained to me, to "realize that a *matai* is his family and not simply the head of his family just like a house is not just a roof, but is also its foundations." This rule of humility applies not only in informal village conferences such as these daily meetings among the older village men, but in the formal meetings of *'āiga* and those formal meetings of *matai* known as the *fono*.

During the morning, older women supervise the younger women in preparing the more substantial mid-morning meal and in pursuing such projects as mat or blind weaving. In villages where they are active, Women's Health Committees often meet in the hours before the morning meal to discuss government health initiatives, to consider village health or other political problems, or to arrange such projects are cleaning up and grooming the church property. Women play a significant and powerful role in Samoan daily life and politics. They are vocal participants in all family and village decisions, in national politics, and in the running of the national education and health clinic system on the islands. While few women hold *matai* titles, their position in *Fa'a Samoa*, and in the web of power and authority in Samoa, is considerable and, in almost all things, equal to that of men. Although women's responsibility for maintaining the grounds of the church may seem a mundane, and even degrading role, it must be understood that caring for the grounds of the church is the women's responsibility because the women of the village effectively control the operations of the church.

At about ten o'clock each morning, the older men and the women, if they are still near their households, sit with their families and enjoy their morning meal. At the same time, the young men working in the plantations stop work and eat a meal of bread and fruit which they have taken with them into the fields. This morning "tea" break is also honoured in businesses and government offices. It is a time of gossip and conversation, of dealing with immediate family problems or planning family activities. It is also a time when relatives and village friends will visit among themselves.

The balance of the morning is spent completing projects started earlier in the day, going to the village store, or driving into the town area to do the day's shopping. In outer villages, this trip to town starts much earlier, governed both by the greater distance, and by the fact businesses shut down between 12 noon and 2 p.m. in the town area. Some people from outer villages will have come to town during the earliest hours of the morning in order to sell their produce at the new market, a major point at which island produce is distributed.

Children leave school at around 1 p.m., before the worst heat of the afternoon, and return home to either play quietly along the village roads or to join their parents or grandparents in an afternoon nap. From about 2 until 4 p.m. the village is almost completely silent, except for the occasional barking dog or soft conversations among children. Most adults remaining in even the central villages of the town area will nap through the worst of the day's heat and the young men working the plantations, having completed most of their work by around 1 p.m., will either return to the village with food they have harvested, or sleep in specially built plantation houses until late in the afternoon.

By four o'clock the village begins to come to life again. Young men back from the fields, or from their cash jobs, perform their household duties again, feeding the pigs, or preparing the male, boiled, portion of the evening meal, before going off to whatever large field is available, to play rugby or the Samoan version of cricket. Young women and teenage girls, when they are not helping prepare the remainder of the evening meal, will visit among themselves, usually with their younger siblings on their laps.

This period of socializing late in the day is interrupted first by the major evening meal, the largest meal eaten on weekdays, and then again by the *sā*, a period of evening prayer. This period of evening prayer is observed to a lesser or greater extent in most villages in Samoa. Often a bell is sounded to mark the beginning and the end of about a half hour of prayer and hymns. During this time, all other activity is supposed to cease in the village. In some villages, the *aumāga* [a loose association of untitled men], or groups of lower ranking *matai,* patrol the village, ensuring that everyone has gone to their respective houses. Fines, in the form of food or cash or labour, but occasionally punishment such as beatings, are levied against violators. This restriction against activity during the *sā* extends to everyone, including people driving along the island roads. In many villages, men patrol the roads at the entrances to the villages, compelling drivers, through the use of large heavy sticks, to stop, and shut off their cars or trucks until the evening prayer is finished. In other villages, young men will hurl large stones at cars travelling during the *sā*. During my stay a controversy arose over several coastal villages blocking the main airport road during evening prayers. Adjacent villages, where enforcement was less stringent, threatened to beat the young men blocking the roads during the prayers. I heard later that the issue was resolved when the stricter villages agreed only to compel drivers to move very slowly through the villages during evening prayers. They continued to block access to other roads in the village, however. A story I heard several times in villages where observance of the *sā* was not very strict recounted how, usually in an immediately adjacent village with which there was some dispute over land or access to water, the rigid maintenance of evening prayers was so strict that on one occasion the villagers actually allowed a house to burn to the ground rather than interrupt their prayers. The implication, always clearly stated, was that while *Fa'a Samoa* was good, sometimes it was better to be modern.

During both the *sā* and the evening meal, small family units are brought together in relative privacy, and all movement throughout the village comes to an almost complete standstill. This is the dignified core of the day's schedule, the sharing of food and the coming together of families in prayer, and it marks the end of the day's formal activities as well. While early evening may be spent visiting or socializing, the few hours following the *sā* until people begin to retire, is a period of constraint and quiet, broken only by the sound of televisions playing martial arts films or groups of young people laughing and singing. In villages in the town area evening socializing may take the form of visits to Apia "night clubs," of which there are several, or of drives in the family's pickup around the streets of the town.

Sundays break the rhythm of labour and rest beginning with the tolling of the church bell at sunrise. Young men in each household have been awake since well before dawn, preparing the *umu*, an earth oven in which the day's major meal, the *to'ana'i*, will be cooked. The preparation of this meal is so important and time consuming, that the Samoan word for Saturday is *aso to'ana'i*, which was explained to me as meaning the day when we begin preparing the Sunday meal. The tolling of the bell at dawn warns them that the *umu* should now be covered, and they should be preparing to attend the first of two church services which will be held that day. Almost everyone in the village will attend one of the churches in the village on Sunday, the only acceptable absences being for illness, or for those members of the household who must remain at home to finish preparation of the Sunday meal. Following the morning church service, senior *matai* and their wives, along with, occasionally, their adult sons and daughters, gather at the home of the pastor of their church for the main Sunday meal, which is served around noon. This meal, whatever the economic condition of the families, churches, or villages, is always extravagant, including as many as 25 different dishes. It is brought to the pastor's house by young men and women from throughout the village, each family in a village contributing a dish to the feast. Individual village families will eat a smaller, but nonetheless elaborate version of this meal, in their own homes at the same time. Following the *to'ana'i*, almost the entire village retires for the remainder of the afternoon. Some families may travel to one of the many beaches which ring the island, but movement and noise inside the village is strictly prohibited.

Late in the afternoon, a smaller contingent of family members attends the afternoon or evening church service, a somewhat shorter version of the morning service. In some villages, there are as many as 10 church services, beginning at dawn and ending late in the night, but the normal pattern of attendance is two services each Sunday. Following the church service, the evening is spent socializing around or between villages. Young people from villages in and around the Apia town area may go into town to one of the two movie theatres showing martial arts and war films, Sunday being these theatres busiest night. Unlike weekday evenings, socializing on Sunday evenings usually continues very late into the evening, the village finally settling into sleep closer to midnight, in contrast to the usual 10 p.m. retirement during the work week.

Idyllic and restful, Samoan village life is remarkable for its similarity throughout the more than 20 villages I visited and stayed in, during my time in Samoa. However, the preceding paragraphs over idealize it, in order to give a sense of the ebb and flow of activity over the course of the day. There is more to daily life, and certainly more to evening activities, than this pastoral picture suggests. The ideal day is one of diminishing activity, such that following the *sā*, the village should be slowly descending into sleep. The day is organized around its still points as objectives, as points in the day to be accomplished. The day is also a time of complex variation, from visits by the *pulenu'u*, the village mayor, who serves as the functional link between the *matai* of the village and the government, to the deliveries of coconuts, by huge dump trucks, from the government plantations. There are fights between groups of boys, village entertainments on the *malae,* and massive ceremonial gatherings for weddings and funerals. Even with these often disruptive variations, daily life in Samoa is remarkable for its stately sameness, whether in the traffic clogged villages of the town area, or the isolated fishing villages of the remote Aleipata district of Upolu.

Stillness and calm, whatever their idyllic qualities, must not obscure the fact village life Samoa is also physically demanding and tiring. In spite of 150 years of influence from more agriculturally advanced sources, subsistence farming in Samoa is still labour intensive and exhausting. It requires patience and skill to bring a crop of taro from its first planting to maturity, and this combination of patience and skill is at the heart of the ideal of strength to which Samoans aspire. While Samoans admire the physical prowess of athletes, in particular their own national rugby team, strength, they will tell you, is not a matter of extremes of power. Rather, strength is measured in terms of endurance. The strong person is not the person who can lift 100 coconuts, although such a feat might be momentarily admired. Instead, the strong person is the person who can lift 10 coconuts 100 times. The loss of strength associated with age is not a decreasing in the power a person can expend, since older men will often perform the same manual tasks as younger ones. Rather, the loss is a loss of endurance. Strength is not a matter of brute power, but of longevity. So the day, however stately and regular, is also a time of great physical exertion by many villagers, a time of real labour and exhaustion. The progress toward the stillness of the *sā*, and the evening that follows, is a progress of fatigue as well as one of cultural ideals.

Where day is an almost stately progression of still points leading to the final still point of the *sā* and the evening meal, night is often an inversion of the stillness of daily life. Night is the time of invisibility and as such, is the time of the greatest privacy, and the greatest unobserved movement. Young people take full advantage of the night, and the enveloping stillness their parents retreat into, to pursue those activities which are most dangerous to the objectives of dignity and stillness in village life. Young men often gather in peer groups, on beaches or bridges, or in night clubs in Apia, to drink beer and fight, and to pursue the young women who spend their evenings travelling the more distant village roads. Night is the time for *ta'a*, roaming, and although calling someone *ta'a* is both an insult and a moral condemnation, implying that the person is unattached and uncontrollable, adults will often tell you that night is the time for young people to be *ta'a* because young people need it to help them grow into full, mature adults. Outside direct control and direct surveillance, village night life includes the socializing of groups singing on the steps of houses, on the one hand, and wandering bands of boys looking for fights, on the other, all in the context of a space of increasing danger, as darkness isolates and hides the villagers from each other. It is this increasing danger and the asociality of the darkness, which encourages practices whose objectives are to draw back the veil of invisibility night brings with it. One such practice, of calling *fā* [a short form of the more formal *tofā*, goodbye] to people passing you in the dark or to cars or trucks passing you on the road, and in particular to calling "goodnight" to people you cannot see and identify, sustains sociality and a simulacrum of visibility even in the concourse of night time travels. "I tell that man walking through my village that I know he is coming by, that he is here in my village, and welcome, and I know him, and his coming through my village" a young man explained to me, "and when I travel somewhere, I call out too, because I want them to know I am a good person passing their house, and not a *ta'a* boy or an *aitu* [evil spirit or being]."

Village life, then, is a repeating pattern of contrasts between stillness and movement, and surveillance and privacy, a balanced, but always tense, antagonism which energizes the village, and sustains its regularity with inherent transgression and ambiguity. Daily village life, simple and calm though it most certainly is, is the site of different types of necessary labour, from the labour of subsistence farming or house maintenance to the labour of drawing outside the still gaze of constant surveillance into the dangerous spaces of darkness and privacy. Bodies circulate in the various spaces of day and night, in calm progress toward quiet and sleep, in the intensive labour of taro and banana patches and pig feeding, or in the spaces of conversation or *ta'a*, when various kinds of bodies connect in pursuit of the balanced articulation of the *aga* of *matai* planning a new road or the *lēaga* of village boys stepping outside the confines of the village and engaging the world in their exploration of the darker spaces outside direct social control.

I began this chapter with a pithy quote from Oscar Wilde, who, as an historical figure, certainly knew his share of contrariness and transgression. I was not being glib in choosing to open with his words. Daily life in Samoa is calm, orderly, even stately. It is also deeply fragmenting, argumentative, and hostile. That is not a contradiction. Indeed, in the logic of Samoans concern with dignity, humility, and strength, it could be no other way. The conceptual logic of daily life in Samoa is structured to both constrain Samoan action and to open spaces for transgression and dispute. But what it also does is create a nexus of fundamental concerns which, when they operate and operate well, resolves contention and transgression. In the years since my first stay in Samoa, not much has changed though everything has certainly changed. That is also not contradictory. The articulation of the pursuit of dignity and accomplishment with the centrality of humility as a core social value requires accommodation, adaptation, and constant revision. In this way then, *Fa'a Samoa* is an ongoing process of absorption and adjustment, argument and negotiation. I once described it to a colleague, accustomed as he was to working in the fractiousness of highland Papua New Guinea, as a kind of authoritarian egalitarianism. The incorporation of still points, oases if you will, in the flux of daily praxis, whether in the calm centre of the *sā*, or in the exigent practicality of children knowing where to play and where to be silent, levels disorder by giving it regularity and direction. Samoa is a riotous revel of smells and noise, of competing demands and insouciant co-operativeness. It is vigorous and often angry. At the same time it is peaceful and steady. I hope the chapters that follow show this more fully than this too brief introductory review can.

I also headed this chapter with a quote from a novel by Naipaul. I arrived in Samoa knowing it well, though in a very literate and literary way. I knew what to expect, where to look, how to understand. What I did not know was the Samoa I knew on arrival was a Samoa embedded in the peculiar pasts we anthropologists create with our writing. It is a past in that it locks in text the specifics of a moment. However, I do not want to lapse into the trite truism that all ethnography is but a fleeting snapshot of an ongoing event, the living processes of a culture in action. As a reader, you know this to be true and need not be insulted by some didactic reminder. What I hoped that quote, and this chapter, would convey to you is a willingness to conspire with me in reading this text outwards to your own knowledgeable pasts, whether a knowledge of Samoa or of your own day-to-day rounds. Think of this chapter, then, as an invitation to see Samoa as my own particular body, my own peculiar histories, and my own specific interests, saw it, while at the same time, reading into the text your own expectations, understandings, and experiences. The world of everyday life is overpopulated with these particularities, and this chapter is one of them. Your reading is another. Taken together, they shape a shifting, and never complete, picture.

And taken together, the regular practices of daily life, and the multiple, and often contentious, understandings of history, form a space within which Samoans constitute their fundamental concerns with dignity, humility, and strength. These three things, taken together into a rhetorical complex, are examples of what Hallpike [1986] describes as "core principles." While his objective was to define central cognitive and conceptual components of a society, echoing Benedict's [1961] earlier model of cultural types, I am deploying these concepts here not as an a priori frame into which I have inserted *Fa'a Samoa*, but instead as key organizing strategies Samoans themselves deploy in making their embodied presence in the world meaningful and effective. The following chapters will explore how these concerns are directly implicated in the ongoing practices of embodiment on which this book focusses. Whether a young boy asking that he be circumcised, a woman avoiding walking in the darker spaces of the bush at night when she is pregnant, or a *matai* accepting a ceremonial cup of *'ava* at an important village meeting, the acts of being in the world through which and because of which good, proper healthy bodies come into being are conditioned and constrained by this tripartite rhetoric of honour and prestige, reticence and modesty, and vigour, stability, and integrity. What I have shown here is the regularity and consistency of daily life, with its built in tensions and transgressions, around which all aspects of *Fa'a Samoa* are focused. It is in these apparently contradictory objectives of stillness and labour, and cooperation and the potential for conflict, that *Fa'a Samoa* is enacted, in its richness and contrariness. Samoans balance, in their daily lives, a complex of opposites, with the ease of a breeze lifting the leaves of a coconut tree in a dance-like synchrony. The following chapters explore particular sites in this process where the body is both an object, and a participant, in this enabling dance.

Chapter 4

Becoming Real: Making Babies into Bodies

Making bodies is work. From conception to birth to the first steps a child takes away from its mother and father, and into the community , the body that is being carried into the social field is being made through the practices of embodiment. I want to explore several points in this enactment which implicate a particularly important moment in embodiment, that is, the moment when we attend to some new body. To do this, in this and the next chapter I will consider the linked processes of reproduction, birth and infancy, and the embodying practices of propriety and restraint. In each case, the body is being marked with basic meanings. The body of the infant, and the body of the foetus before it, are being assigned values, and probed for meanings drawn from particular experiences and understandings of proper body form and movement. This probing is a key embodying strategy which initiates a life long process of sustaining a proper body.

Writing about matters which Samoans are often hesitant to speak about, and this applies most particularly to questions of sex and birth, is difficult, in part because the material needs to be linked from a wide range of informants, often revealed in tiny bits and pieces. It is also difficult because the act of writing, as a public act, violates fundamental rules of propriety and modesty, and as such, violates certain fundamental aspects of Samoan embodiment itself. I realized very early in my fieldwork that what I was being told was often in strict and very hushed confidence, the confidence of, in some cases intimates, and in others the confidence of protecting misimpressions by telling me things which, though normally private, needed to be explained to ensure my understandings were as thorough as possible. Material throughout this section on pregnancy and the development of the foetus is drawn extensively from conversations with older women, beyond their reproductive years, who felt they could reasonably and without undue embarrassment speak with me about matters women, under normal circumstances, do not speak about, even with their husbands.

I want to stress however that this embarrassment is not a function of modesty or repression, though each has been insinuated into issues of sex and sexuality in Samoa. The embarrassment expresses the potentially dangerous and divisive aspects of sex and reproduction for Samoans. Sex, and in particular, sex between husband and wife, is the site of the most fundamental of Samoan social obligations, the reproduction of *Fa'a Samoa* through the reproduction of meaningful Samoan bodies. This obligation makes sex socially dangerous, Because so much depends on its success.

In writing about explications of impregnation and foetal development, I want to issue a warning. What follows is not to be taken as a "traditional" model of pregnancy in contrast to some more bio-medical one. As I've noted, Samoans are loathe to discuss these matters in anything but euphemism or by allusion, which makes understanding intimate organic processes difficult. But more important, the details I am about to outline must not be read as either quaint or as generally shared. They are no more quaint than the over 200 explanations of gestation I have collected from children, adolescents, and adults in two ongoing studies of individual biological models and health seeking behaviour in Ontario, Canada.[1] What follows is a composite of several accounts in order to outline the principles of balance, propriety, and organic flow which characterize Samoan biological models as they relate to pregnancy, inheritability of traits, and the process of infant growth and socialization. It is only in principle, and not in detail, that it is possible to say these ideas are generally shared. This is true of all forms of cultural knowledge, after all. Pealing back the layers of individual detail, however, reveals that the core notions of the combination of body fluids, and the integral connection between propriety and foetal and infant health are shared, though sometimes quite inarticulately. Though there is great variety in the details of the many accounts of pregnancy I heard, the basic melody remains the same. What I hope the reader takes from the discussion below is a sense of the connection between these often variable ideas about mechanical detail and larger concerns with order and propriety, rather than passing judgement on how misguided this explanation of pregnancy appears to be, though this always remains a substantial and unavoidable risk whenever anthropologists write about local knowledge, and in this case, local biologies.

Genital body fluids are not defined as either powerful or polluting by Samoans. In contrast, genital body fluids are often dangerous or sacred substances throughout Melanesia [see, for example, Herdt 1999, 1981; Meigs 1983; Jorgensen 1983]. Indeed, Samoans are remarkably quiet about semen and menses, and no efforts are made to conserve semen, and menstruation, while embarassing and deeply private because of its association with marital sex and pregnancy, is not ritualized or secret.[2] There are no restrictions, other than those on speaking openly about them, on touching or seeing either semen or menstrual blood. I should note however, that while women could and did speak with some candour about menstruation, though in ways always circumscribed by both privacy and embarrassment, men found talking about semen, either their own or semen in general, troublesome. However, what became clear to me during the collection of sexual histories from men of various ages is that the embarrassment is more closely connected to the way discussion of semen draws attention to a mans penis than some embarrassment about the substance itself. Making the penis visible, even in conversation, is, for many Samoan men, more fraught with embarrassment than discussing what it is the penis is used for.

There are also no menstrual purifying or protecting practices, and no prohibitions on sexual activity during menses, in contrast to the often complex rules and prohibitions surrounding menstruation and female pollution found not only in the Pacific but throughout the world, not excluding our own clouded and euphemized practices surrounding "the curse" [see, for example, Buckley and Gottlieb 1988]. While Fitzgerald [1989] suggests that menstrual blood may have been considered polluting in pre-European Samoa, today most Samoans find this idea either humorous, or evidence of the "stupid ideas" that may have been current prior to the Christianization of Samoa. Rather, genital body fluids are treated as practical substances, like building materials in a house, and their relationship to impregnation is understood solely in terms of a biology of combinations.

Through sexual intercourse, semen travels into the area around the *to'ala*, or stomach heart, an organ which normally resides in the abdominal cavity slightly below the sternum. An open space around this organ, known as the *fa'aautagata* [roughly "to cause a person, carried here, to flow from this place"], is the location for the combination of semen and the blood of the mother which results in the development of the foetus [*tama fafano*, literally "non-adult person [*tama*] in a bowl" [*fafano*]]. Although all the dictionaries I consulted give womb as the translation for *fa'aautagata*, it was never clear to me whether my informants were speaking of an organ, in the sense in which we use the term, or were simply referring to a place in the abdomen. Most people, when asked to translate *fa'aautagata* into English as they understood it, adopted variations of the phrase "the place where babies come from" or "the place where babies are made." Since the infix "au" has two connotations—to carry and to flow, as in a current—simply translating this in the English sense of womb misses the conceptual richness contained in the Samoan word.

In impregnation, semen [*si*] provides white body substances such as bones, muscle, fat and skin. Blood from the mother provides the developing baby not only with blood, but also with the soft organs both inside the body, such as the liver or spleen, as well as, and perhaps most importantly, organs which connect the body to the outside world, such as the eyes or the tongue. Additional substances needed for the development of these body components is provided by the food the pregnant mother eats, including an increase in the amount of white, boiled, male food such as taro or bananas and especially, rice.[3] A relationship of combining substances of like colour conjoins with a sense of the practical complementarity of male and female body substances, creating the initial combination of substances from which the foetus develops. While linguistically marked such that one may only use the polite words for both blood [*toto*] and semen [*si*] when speaking of pregnancy and birth, rather than words from the more vernacular vocabulary [*gafa*, blood and *pā*, to explode, respectively], this does not mark these substances as special. Pregnancy may only be spoken of in polite terms, out of modesty rather than mystification. The process is not special, but talking about it is circumscribed, because so much social capital and social obligation is invested in it.

Another feature of this combination of male and female substances, and the tissues they produce, relates to the question of sexing. That men's muscle tissue provides the building blocks for the muscle tissue of the foetus is important because it introduces a certain ambiguity about gender and sexing at the very beginning of the emergence of a functional Samoan body. Both the penis and the vagina are, conceptually, muscles. Both the penis and the vagina are, conceptually, male organs, since they are examples of male substance rendered into different practical forms. This ambiguity over what we consider to be core identifying features of bodies which are defined by Samoans as the same thing in different forms sites the process of sexing bodies somewhere other than solely on the surface of the body itself. Genitals are not sufficient to determine the sex of an individual. The sexing of persons, which is socialized during middle childhood, is derived from what is done with bodies as a whole, rather than from some innate sexing quality of the genitals alone.[4]

The admixture of semen and blood, derived as they are from the parent's two bodies, is the process by which physical attributes from both parents combine in the physical form of the emerging baby.[5] Although both men and women have bones and fat, as well as internal red organs, those of men are stronger, and more valuable for healthy foetal development. Equally, women and men share almost all the same internal organs, but women's internal organs are considered stronger because women are subject to fewer injuries and stresses on these organs from heavy labour. Women's organs are also protected by a substantial layer of fat which does not develop in men until much later in life. As well, both men and women explained to me that menstruation in women ensured that women's blood was always clean and strong.

Heat triggers the combination of semen and female blood, and Samoans consider the sweat raised during sexual intercourse to be evidence of sufficient internal heat in the woman to provide the agitation needed to combine the male and female substances. The action of sex, with its stimulation of the interior of the woman's body, which is evidenced by her sexual pleasure, creates a turbulence in the womb by which the semen and blood are brought together and combined. This turbulence may take several minutes, and may last for as long as several hours, women often reporting agitated disturbances in their abdomen for some time after intercourse. However, no special precautions are taken to either sustain this turbulence, or to protect the woman in any way while this combination is taking place. Many Samoans who spoke with me about pregnancy have taken up the outlines of the egg and sperm model of impregnation, but only to the extent that they understand the components of the foetal egg, based on the egg of chickens, as the thing produced by the combination of semen [the white] and blood [the yolk]. One day, Mele, an 80-year-old great-great grandmother explained to me how, when she learned about the foetal egg, she realized just why Samoa is named Samoa, which is translated by some as "sacred chicken," but which she suggested might mean "sacred egg." For her, this proved beyond argument that "family is Samoa, everything else is *lēaga*, evil, not of God." While many of my Samoan informants were familiar with sperm, and had even seen photographs of these organisms, there was no organized change to the combination model of impregnation, and no formal ascription of a role to the sperm in this process. Rather, as one person told me, "maybe sperm move around and mix the semen and blood together."

Neither semen nor blood is considered to be finite, so the failure of one attempt at impregnation is not a concern. Indeed, repeated acts of intercourse throughout the pregnancy are understood to either help sustain the pregnancy by repeated agitations of the womb, or to ensure that there is a sufficient supply of semen to continue to work in combination with the mother's blood. The only restriction on sex during pregnancy is a practical one. Husbands and wives abstain from genital sex in the later months because it is uncomfortable, and not because it is dangerous.

Pregnancy fulfils a central social imperative for Samoans, the creation of families. The polite phrase for sexual intercourse, *fai'āiga*, translates quite literally as "making families," expressed in its other uses such as "to eat a meal as a family" or "to live together as a family," all three being aspects of making families to my Samoan informants. Sexual arousal and desire is inseparable from Samoans' knowledge about what the substances they combine produce. Sexual desire, expressed in the regular sex lives of husbands and wives, writes social obligation with the genitals, and sexual pleasure is defined at least in part as deriving from a recognition of the "family making" purpose of sex. While I am talking, at this point, about heterosexual sex, I am not talking about heterosexuality, not about the platitudinous connection between sex and procreation advocated by some religious groups, particularly in North America—a connection they see as morally true and natural, to the exclusion of others. *Fai'āiga* is not a concern with heterosexuality, but with family and children, and it does not exclude sex acts so much as place a moral and communal obligation on all sexuality. This functional aspect of marital sex, conjoining a vigourous and passionate enjoyment of sex with an equally vigourous and passionate concern for "making children," is one of the reasons Mead [1961], in her study of Samoan adolescence and sexual mores, failed to recognize that what appears on the surface to be a sensual and liberated sexual pursuit is, in actual practice, heavily mandated and formalized around considerations of social order and obligation. Ejaculation, orgasm, and the other sensual pleasures which attach to sex fulfil sociality and are governed, not only by a concern for pleasure, but for social harmony and moral obligation. As I noted above, sex is the location where social reproduction is at its most intense. It is understandable Mead missed the complex regulation and concern which sex entails on individual Samoans since, after all, she was almost wholly interested in psychological traits which kind of analysis could not but fail to notice the way sex in Samoa is both a deeply private and intensively public act.

Under normal circumstances, pregnancy, once recognized, is announced throughout the 'āiga and village. Only where an unmarried girl or woman becomes pregnant without prospects either of formal marriage or defacto union with the father is pregnancy kept secret. Indeed, in an instance in one village where I lived, a young woman's pregnancy was kept hidden until the early morning when I was wakened to drive her to the National Hospital to give birth. Asking me to drive her and her daughter to the hospital was the final act of secrecy, since Siluga, the new baby's grandmother, told me that she had come to get me to drive because she knew that *palagi* do not gossip. However, because defacto marriages [often called traditional Samoan marriages by my informants], which involve little more than an announcement that the couple intends to live as man and wife, are so readily entered into and abrogated, hidden pregnancies are quite rare. In villages where surveillance is so intense that the fact a couple is having sex at all is rarely a private matter, pregnancies are important because they proclaim the couple is meeting their responsibility in the important master process of creating families.

The progress of pregnancy is generally smooth, with limited restrictions placed on the mother during the course of her term. There are practical prohibitions against dangerous activities, such as climbing or carrying heavy loads, or any activity which could result in a fall and the dislodging of the foetus causing miscarriage [*fafano*, empty bowl]. The expectant mother is not treated with any particular deference or consideration other than being exempted from this heavy labour. Pregnancy, *ma'ito*, is conceptually at least an illness in contemporary practice, but not in the sense of either risk or disease. My informants explained to me that *ma'ito* refers to the fact that pregnant women are weaker, less capable of daily work obligations and likely to be less social because of fatigue or such symptoms as nausea or muscular discomfort. Neither Pratt's 19th century dictionary, nor Milner's 20th century text, based on data from the 1940's and 1950's, give the word *ma'ito* [*ma'i*, illness and *to*, to be pregnant], listing only the word *to*. The attachment of the concepts surrounding illness to pregnancy would appear to be of recent vintage, borne out not only by the linguistic evidence, but by comments by one of my older female informants such as "today women are sick and not pregnant. Every time a baby is coming women get sick and lazy, not like when my mother just worked and worked and did not care until the time came for the baby to be born." In general, most women I spoke with reported that the progress of their pregnancies was physically uneventful and that delivery was easy, whether attended by a healer experienced in *fa'atosaga* [traditional midwifery], or by a doctor in the National Hospital.

However, the progress of foetal development does obligate cautions on the part of the mother and those around her. The foetus is, from the point of the combination of semen and blood, considered to be intimately attached to the mother's body, such that whatever the mother's body is exposed to and whatever the mother's body engages in, directly affects the development and form of the foetus. Anything which adversely affects this accumulative development, either by interfering with the acquisition of mass or obstructing the building up of appropriate tissues in their appropriate locations, is avoided.

Such things as excessive cold or excessive heat, both considered major causes of illness by Samoans, need to be avoided. Extreme cold could cause the child's skin to pucker, resulting in the child being born with mottled or pock-marked skin, while extreme heat could cause the child's skin to become inflamed and weakened, since heat thins the skin. Sudden changes in temperature, as well as sudden movements or loud noises, must be avoided, because their startling affect on the mother transfers directly to the foetus. A mother who is repeatedly startled or frightened during pregnancy will likely have a child who cries a great deal and is either very shy or very easily frightened. Changes in social relations which effect the mother by frightening or angering her are also avoided. Pregnant women are excused from participating in discussions of *'āiga* or village disputes, and arguments are abruptly halted should a pregnant woman come near the arguers. Finally, husbands defer to their wife's wishes more readily during pregnancy, again to avoid angering or upsetting them, and thus effecting the temperament of the child. This deference does not extend to avoidance of sexual relations during pregnancy, since additional semen, as well as additional physical agitation of the abdomen is considered useful for the proper and complete mixing of tissue producing substances during foetal development.

Other sorts of precautions are followed during pregnancy, again high-lighting the homologous connection between the body of the mother and the foetal child. Pregnant women avoid travelling alone at night, because to do otherwise would put them at risk from attack by *aitu*, often malicious spirit beings. These attacks are not mystical in nature. Rather, *aitu* enjoy either frightening women or tripping them capriciously, which endangers the child's temperamental development, or may induce a miscarriage or premature delivery. Pregnant women will avoid completely locations where *aitu* are known to live. For example, the small Papasea gorge just south of Vaimoso has a well known rock slide and swimming hole which people travel to from around the islands. However, it is also known to be the home of a particularly vicious *aitu* known as Saumaiafe. Pregnant women will not only not visit the Papasea sliding rocks during pregnancy, but will avoid even travelling near the village of Papasea itself, or bathing in the river which feeds through this small gorge.

As well as avoiding sites where *aitu* are likely to be encountered, women will take precautions, when they sleep, to protect themselves from *aitu* attack which may take two different forms. The first involves direct attacks on the mother, usually in the form of kicking her, or pulling her hair. To prevent this, pregnant women try to sleep between at least two other persons, increasing the likelihood that one of their sleeping partners will be awakened by the *aitu*'s presence, and be able to ward it off. The other form of attack involves direct attack on the foetus, by either kicking the mother's abdomen or entering the *fa'aautagata* [womb-place] through the vagina, mouth or armpit, and attacking the foetus, breaking its bones, or twisting its muscles. Children born with broken bones or distorted heads are understood to have been victims of *aitu* attack during gestation.

Attacks on women while walking alone at night are arbitrary, reflecting the *aitu*'s malicious and more often than not capricious nature. Attacks on sleeping pregnant women are more troublesome because they are indications of some serious problem in *'āiga* relations. Direct intended attacks by *aitu* most often result from conflicts between *'āiga* members, between residents of related villages, or as a result of some inappropriate or insulting behaviour by the mother, or a member of her *'āiga*, either toward some ancestor, or toward some specific *aitu*. When an attack is known to have occurred, steps are taken to resolve the conflict. When the effect of the attack is not known until after delivery, action will be taken to appease the offended *aitu* and, at the same, the infant will be treated with massage and herbal cures in an effort to repair the damage the *aitu* may have done.

If *aitu* can attack the infant through the mother's body, accidental behaviours by the mother can also affect the progress and outcome of the foetus's physical development [MacPherson and MacPherson 1990:186;

Neitch and Neitch 1974]. Certain foods need to be avoided because they may affect the child. Octopus, for example, may cause the child to be born with rashes, or to suffer them throughout its life. A mother wearing items around her neck can cause the child to become tied up in the umbilical cord. A pregnant woman placing items behind her ears can cause the child's ears to be malformed, while a mother using her teeth to tear either food, or thread in sewing, can cause the child's teeth to protrude or cause tears in the sides of the lips of the foetus's mouth. Not walking upright can lead to stooping in the child, while walking too quickly can cause the child's legs to overdevelop, making delivery, and learning to walk, difficult. What is common to all of these is a direct relationship between the body of the foetus and the mother's body. The foetus and the mother, as bodies, are inseparable. Changes in one are mirrored in changes in the other. A foetus which is developing malformed limbs may manifest itself in the mother's arms and legs, while developing malformations in the mouth or lips may be expressed in the face of the mother. In one case, a woman noted for her smile complained that it was becoming increasingly difficult for her to open her mouth and expose her teeth at all. A Samoan healer examined the position of the infant in the *fa'aautagata* and determined that the child's head was too large and that its face was being pressed against the wall of the mother's abdomen. Massage repositioned the foetus in a more appropriate orientation and the mother's facial constrictions were relieved.

The notion of the homologous relationship between mother and foetus extends to the father as well. It is possible for both the mother and father to pass along what might be called "personality" traits to the foetus through the mixture of semen and maternal blood. However, this heritability of traits is explicitly physical in nature rather than cognitive or psychological. Certain character attributes such as patience, calmness, a tendency to anger easily and so on are directly related to the size, functioning and positioning of internal organs such as the *to'ala*. It is the character of these organs which is inherited, and not the consequential temperaments and traits. This is perhaps best captured in the complement paid to someone considered wise and patient—she has a strong heart, Samoans will say. They mean that literally, and not metaphorically.

Massage and dietary advice are the primary forms of obstetric care, whether received from a Samoan healer, from a doctor at the National Hospital, or from a nurse at a village health clinic. Samoan healers monitor changes in mass in the woman's abdomen through probing massage, and their treatment during the pregnancy consists mostly of correcting the foetal orientation, or adjusting the mother's internal organs. Both ensure an easy passage for the foetus at birth and keep the mother's bladder and bowels moving freely to avoid potentially dangerous obstructions. Medical doctors from the hospital or local clinics, in co-operation with village women's health committees, provide prenatal care in the form of dietary advice and supplements, as well as some formal education about infant care. The general thrust of pre-natal care is to keep the mother comfortable, to ensure she avoids unnecessary risks, and to monitor the development of body mass in the foetus, objectives which are shared by both the traditional midwife and the Western trained medical personnel. This often means that pregnant women avail themselves of both types of service interchangeably, depending on which is more convenient at a given moment in the progress of their pregnancy.

Labour and delivery, whether in the village under the care of a healer experienced in *fa'atosaga* [midwifery], or in the hospital under Western medical supervision, should include the complete expulsion of all materials related to the pregnancy. Delivery is not thought to be complete until all the cellular debris has been expunged from the "womb" and the cervix has returned to normal. Particular care is taken to prevent vaginal prolapse, *ma'i lalovasa*, or the displacement of the internal organs, which can result from the pressure the *to'ala* [stomach heart] exerts on the foetus to help with its delivery. Massage and rest following pregnancy ensure a quick return to fertility.

Infant health, like foetal health, is understood in terms of the continued accumulation of appropriate tissue mass. Average birth weight in Samoa is approximately 3.5 kg, and is in the mid-range of averages in world populations [Bindon and Zansky 1986:224-225]. However, 12 month weight gain in Samoa is rapid and considerable, average 12 month weight for both boys and girls being around 10.5 kgs [p.246]. While infancy is normally a period of "rapid hyperplastic growth," Samoan infants' weight gain in the first months of life is equal to, or greater than the 75th percentile average for American children [p.227]. The child is breast-fed, fed infant formula provided by the women's health committee, and fed increasing quantities of white food, especially boiled rice. An increase in bottle-feeding of babies in American Samoa has led to an increase in average weight gain among infants [p.236], which Bindon and Zansky suggest combines with a possible genetic predisposition toward obesity in later life.

At the same time, the mother eats large amounts of white starch foods in order to maintain her weight. The health of the mother, observable in both her return to normal day to day activities, and in the maintenance of her weight, is tied to the health of the child. Illness in the mother during the first year of her infant's life often requires curative treatment of both the mother and the baby.

The child should grow rapidly during the first year of life and should be alert and active, seeking out human contact and demonstrating a curiosity about the world around it. As well, infant death is a serious concern for Samoan mothers. Bannister et al. [1978], found a decline in infant mortality in Samoa, from about 100 per 100,000 in 1950 to about 70 per 100,000 in 1970 [cited in Harbison 1986:73]. Infant mortality was estimated at 50/100,000 in 1989 [per.comm. Samoa Department of Statistics] based on data for the period between 1984 and 1986. This compares with Canada, at about 60/100,000, and the United States, at about 90/100,000, for the same period. However, these estimates are based on questionable birth and death registration data. Both inaccuracies in the data collection systems employed over the course of this century, and Samoan's tendency to not consistently report births and deaths, have contributed to limitations on most health statistics in Samoa. Most older women with large families, however, told me they had lost at least one child in infancy, while younger mothers fully expected that at least one of their babies would die in its first year. One protection against sudden death of an infant is to keep the baby in the company of caregivers at all times. From very early on, the child is carried by the mother or her older children, when they go to perform work around the village, or to travel into town or to other villages. It is almost always held facing away from the bearer and toward what is happening around them. While protecting the child from extremes of heat and cold, no other substantial effort is made to coddle the baby. It becomes an active body in the meaningful life of the village, and the wider community, almost from the day of its birth [Ochs 1988:85]. Its progress in weight gain, developing alertness, and social skills, are closely observed and commented on by all who come into contact with it. Its body is a constant focus of attention by friends and relatives, its weight, feces, and vomit, noted and discussed. Fluids must move through the body and should not be obstructed or hampered in their flow. Feces, for example, must be syrupy and easily passed, evidence of properly working digestion and breathing. All of the infants' activities are monitored and observed. Particular attention is paid to the strength of its crying and the loudness of its voice. The gathering strength of its limbs is encouraged with games, such as placing small long objects in the infant's hand and then trying to pull them away.

During the first several months, the infant is spoken to constantly, a combination of nonsense sounds, often delivered in a sing-song voice by both men and women, and simple commands such as "stop," "quiet" and "stand still." Everyone in the household is involved in caring for the infant, with the father doing the least, although he remains an active caregiver [Ochs 1988:78-80]. From early on the child is encouraged to sleep at the same time adults sleep and be awake when adults are normally awake [Mead 1961]. Most women told me their babies slept through the night within several weeks of being born, and my own experience in households with infants confirms this.

From 12 months onward, a healthy baby, most easily identified as a very large and very loud baby, begins its physical transition to the status

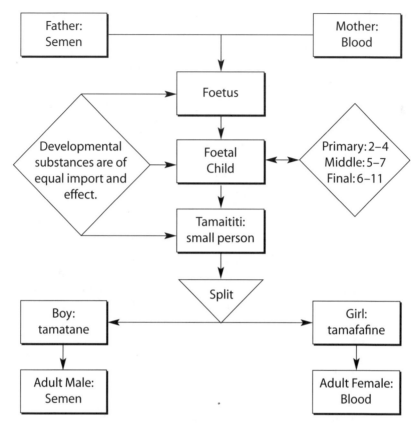

Figure 4.1 The stages of growth from foetus to adult,
showing the relative predominance of "sexed" substances.

of child. This involves certain physical changes. Expectations of noise and movement become inverted as the process of socialization into appropriate body language and body style begins. The first 12 months of life can be thought of as continuing the process of gestation post-partum, in that the expectation of massive weight gain is encouraged throughout this period through overfeeding. The infant remains a foetus in its physical care, and its progress towards childhood remains closely attached to its mother's body and health. The *tamameamea* [child-gift thing] remains special and distinctive during its first year, encouraged in excesses while at the same time encouraged in its attachment to others. Never left alone, fed on demand, prompted to be hyper-active and often annoyingly loud, the infant is being lead into socially meaningful presence.

The destination of this year of attentive indulgence is a transition toward a new set of expectations about good and proper bodies, and the steady progress toward mature status both as bodies and as persons. There are stages to this process, where the infant progresses from being a kind of foetal child—up to about age 4 or so—and then through subsequent phases of middle and final childhood ending at around age 12. During this period, the word most often used for a child is *tamaititi*, or small person. It is generic, and is applied to both boys and girls. From about 12 onward, however, the generic name is replaced by sexed words—*tamatane*, *tamafafine*—small or incomplete male or female—and *fa'afafine* [the third sex, biological male but socially some other sex.][6] At marriage, boys and girls are referred to as either *tane* or *tama*, male and female respectively, this including recently married *fa'afafine*. It is the emergence of explicit sexing after childhood, which is of key importance because it is tied to the increasing importance of one body substance over another. Figure 4.1 shows the stages of development of from foetus to adult. Up to about 12 years of age, blood and semen are equally present and equally important in their development roles in the growth of the childs body. But at about age 12, not coincidentally the period around which time secondary physical sexual characteristics begin to emerge, semen and blood begin to take on differential degrees of importance in the fuller growth of biologically male and female bodies. What is most telling, however, is that this is a biological form of sexing which is distinctive from the embodied process of sexing which does not rely on body form as a marker of sex. Samoans distinguish explicitly between bodies as things governed by inscrutable rules of process and mechanics, and bodies as things which have and generate meaning in the social field. That is, while bodies are mechanically sexed by the play of sexing substances, semen and blood, this is not a constraint or determining characteristic of the bodies ultimate meaning. That meaning is engaged through other processes in which bodies in the world are divided up into generic types, that is through the process of embodiment rather than those of biology. This process begins earlier than the ultimate biological division which begins to occur during adolescence, with boys through circumcision, and with the more stringent application of rules of genital modesty on girls, but it is not until adolescence that formal sexing in marked in language consistently. What this suggests is that the body is an unfinished project as an organic object for more than a decade after the birth of a child. It is not so much that it is changing as it is continuing to emerge, to come into existence. As such, the body of the growing child is engaged in both a strategy of coming into full social being, and an ongoing gestation as it continues its process of meaningful development.

The ideal body style in Samoa is a combination of mass, strength, and stillness. The good and proper Samoan body is one which is imposing in its pure physical presence, but neither particularly active nor in any way domineering. That is to say, the good and proper body, is large and silent, moves slowly, but with steady and capable purpose, and never imposes itself by displays of specialness or distinction. This inverts the expectations of the good infant body. With the transition to childhood, the body of the child has now become socially informed and is now part of the process of constituting the social field. The training of the body in seemliness and suitability marks the emergence of the baby as a social being. Sione, a mother of 11 living children, one afternoon, explained it this way:

> When a baby is born, it has to be shown everything, made to see everything and do everything because that is the only way it can know what the things are in the world that it must know, and so we don't punish babies and we won't yell at them and we like to see them crying and screaming and moving. We take them everywhere so they can see everything and then, later, when they are older, we can teach them what all the things they have seen, what they mean, and then we can teach them to be quiet.

* * *

In the earliest stages of embodiment, when the infant is beginning to be attended to as a body by those around it, the body is being enacted as socially meaningful, given social presence. Through the gaze of its caregivers, the probing touch of relatives and friends caressing and pinching and holding it, the body of the infant, and the infant's emerging awareness of itself as a socially meaningful body, are in transition. The restraint of parental care, from early toileting, cleaning, and feeding, to games played with body parts, engages the infant's body in a process of transformation initiated by the observers around it. Attention begins, in Samoa, with the singular qualities of the particular infant's body being measured against a set of fixed, general, expectations about how and when bodies will grow, move, and develop. The locus of attention, on the surface of the body, and on what can be observed and directly interpreted, sets the ground for the child's emerging awareness of itself as a thing that can be attended to, directing its own gaze and probing interpretation, by example, to attend to its skin, scent, and body products.

Equally important, however, the focus of attention, which encompasses not only the infant, but also the mother, and her relationships, establishes a different aspect of the ground of embodiment, which begins to direct the child's experience of its body in terms of how it is inexorably connected to the other bodies around it. In essence, the infant discovers the boundaries of its body, through the attention of others to its bodily processes. And in discovering that bodily boundary, begins to enact through its body the web of interconnection — seeing and being seen, doing and being done to and so on—which deploys its social self as an embodied praxis linking the emergent borders of the physical body indivisibly with the community of other bodies through which the infant has begun to navigate. This is not simply a matter of knowing by experience the difference between me/not me but slowly coming to understand that what I am as a real organic object acting in and on the world is the process of reconciling and negotiating, over and over, the fluidity and permeability of that boundary. The process of being attended to, and coming to know how to attend to and so make the world around it, produces not so much an ego object, though the core embodied experience is the recognition of "my" body as a physical thing [Winnicott 1986]. Rather, the processes of attention and attending initiate a life long ego process in which the body is both a product and tool. The infant learns, through the coming into being of its body as a social object, that it is always in a state of transition between thing and action. It is embodying the world its body engages as both a cause and effect.

Childhood, *aso fa'a tamaititi*, the "days of making a small person," is a period of extensive socialization and training. Throughout this period, the foetal child of the first year of life becomes fully engaged, as a participant, in its community, and in the enactment of its body as a part of that community. The child is beginning the long progress toward maturity and adulthood. It is a progress marked by the child's socialization into propriety and appropriate body presence, and most particularly by its socialization into a particular manner of attending to itself and the bodies around it. Childhood involves, among its many lessons, learning to be a body, and it is to that process of embodying propriety—teaching children to be quiet—that I now turn.

Chapter 5

Embodying Moral Orders: Space, Modesty, and Eating

At the end of the last chapter I spoke of the process of recognition through which the body of the infant is attended to as a socially meaningful thing by those around it. This process forms the foundation on which the child begins to learn the subjective exigencies through which embodiment is accomplished. In this chapter, I will focus on selected aspects of socialization, through which the child becomes complicit in the process of embodiment and meaning as an active participant. Through socialization of the child's body practice it learns to account for its presence and abilities in the world. This learning how to account for our physical presence is central to embodiment, because it is through accounting for the world, and one's presence in it, that the body can be deployed as a socially meaningful act. At the same time, the process of embodiment needs to be understood as constitutive of that account of the world, inseparable from it. The body socialized is also a body socializing the world it moves in and around. By learning how to sit in church, or the proper way to hold and chew its food, the child begins to use its body to constitute the social space in which it lives.

Where infant socialization can be described as a process of marking the salient features on the childs embodied map of the world with boundaries and with an outward focus which highlights the importance of observing and being observed as aspects of embodied presence, socialization of children becomes most explicitly a collaboration in which the child becomes a fully social body by giving up ownership of its boundaries and more fully siting its embodied praxis in the contingent demands of multiple engagements between organic realities and processes of self consciousness and collaboration. In these early years of socialization, the child disowns itself as a discrete object as it becomes an object enmeshed in the social landscape. While the boundaries between me and not me I spoke of in the previous chapter remain, they become less and less fixed. It is perhaps ironic that the period of the greatest physical helplessness, infancy, is also the period during which the child has the greatest ownership and control of its body as a thing. In the years of childhood socialization, it will give up that ownership as its body becomes more socially "real" and less or-

91

ganically "fixed" in its active presence, manipulation, and construction of its embodied social world.

Heston was 4 years old in 1991, the second youngest son of the daughter of a ranking *matai*. He was born in Hawai'i, where his parents had lived for fifteen years. At age 3, Mafa, his mother, had brought him to Samoa, and had left him in the care of his grandparents in order that he could grow up learning to be a "good and strong Samoan." Heston was sickly, suffering from a susceptibility to bronchial infection labelled by those around him as asthma. He had been a very small baby, and in his second and third years, his growth had been markedly stunted and slow. "He needs to be in Samoa," Mafa explained, "because he needs to get a strong body from growing up as a Samoan boy."

Samoans living overseas, as part of the ring of extended kinship which extends to New Zealand and Australia in the south and, to the north, to Fiji, Hawai'i and California, often characterize Samoa as the source of their health and strength. Samoans who become ill while living overseas, often return to Samoa to recover. De facto adoptions of Samoan children born overseas by relatives living in Samoa is quite common [Kallen 1982]. These adoptions have two main objectives, one focused on the child qua child, and the other on the extended family of which the child is a member. Returning a child to Samoa engages *Fa'a Samoa* itself as a tutor through which the child learns the good and proper way to be Samoan and to have a good and proper Samoan body. "Overseas children are too cheeky and too weak," I was told. "They need the air and the work and family in Samoa to make them good so they can grow up to be real, you know, finished, whole Samoans."[1] At the same time, de facto transfer of children from their overseas parents to Samoan relatives adds additional assistance and support to the pool of family labour. "Children are their parent's arms and legs," Pai, my Samoan mother, would remind me whenever I would ask her about how her own children had learned to perform their household duties. Caring for children is also a key component of youthfulness and full community participation. As one great-grandmother told me, "until my children have no more children, I am still young because I am still a mother."

Children are of central importance in Samoan life because "they are our future, when they will care for old men and women, and they are our present because teaching *Fa'a Samoa* is how *Fa'a Samoa* stays alive and keeps alive." The process of socializing children begins shortly after birth, when infants are brought with adults, or other caregivers, to all events in the village, rather than being isolated in protected nurseries. It is continuous, and becomes something which the child learns to participate in as well. They are always held facing outward, their gaze directed toward the activity around them, their gaze drawing the gaze of those around them inward to attend to their presence. This circular relationship between being socialized, and socializing the world around one, is accomplished most directly in the way a child learns to enact a proper body in his or her daily practices.

Much has been written about childrearing in Samoa, most often from the perspective of the inculcation of stringent social control [Freeman 1984] or the absence of efforts to impose control [Mead 1961, 1969]. What both these authors have failed to take into account is that the objective of socialization in Samoa is not comparable to that in the societies from which these researchers came. Where North American socialization, for example, is about learning to control urges, and to postpone gratification, Samoan socialization is about learning to direct urges and pursue gratification in a manner which is both proper in the sense of modest and humble, and exploratory. Both Freeman and Mead, as Ochs [1988;147-148] notes, were looking for domination and control, in some absolute and punishing form. Because of this, they missed the subtlety of Samoan socialization, which has as its objective not domination, but co-operation, and not submission but support. Learning appropriate body function contributes to this process in subtle ways.

Samoans experience most body functions as being discrete processes, although the details of their biological modelling are different from Western scientific biology. This includes, for Samoans, their experience of body functions as always undergoing development, transformation, and improvement. These developments in the major body functions are seen as progressive rather than regressive or degrading. Where North American toilet training, for example, involves learning not to defecate, and to control and disguise body function, Samoan toilet training is about learning to defecate in an appropriate and healthy manner. Samoan children do not learn to stop up their bowels, they learn how to keep them flowing.

There are four areas of body function in Samoan biology: the excretory, the gustatory, the respiratory, and the cognitive/sensory. I will restrict my discussion below to only the first two, since the principles of appropriate flow of body substances is, in these areas, most directly related to the enactment of dignity. Each set of body processes progresses through development from excess to calm restraint, as the child grows during its *aso fa'a tamaititi* [childhood period] into young adult and then adult status. The period of excess is characterized as a period of inadequacy of function, rather than one of lack of control. The excretory functions exemplify this.

Little or no effort is taken to impose urinary and bowel control on infants or very young children. It was not unusual to see a toddler, having just learned to walk, stop to defecate in the middle of the *malae*, or to urinate outside the door of its *fale*. However, what Mead [1961:18-20] saw as a lack of control of children, became on questioning my informants, a matter of biology. As I noted in the last chapter, foetal development continues post-partum for at least the first year and sometimes slightly later, if an infant has not gained sufficient weight to be considered healthy. During this time, the internal organs and the paths along which body substances are travelling are still growing and developing. To interfere with the excretory processes risks interfering with, or obstructing the complete and healthy formation of these organs. The ultimate and healthy form of the excretory pathways is one of easy and smooth flow. Any interference which would jeopardize this is avoided, not only in children, but in adult life as well. The use of mild purgatives, and of massage to assist infants and young children whose bowels or bladder do not appear to be developing properly because they are not sufficiently productive, is quite common. Most mothers know the appropriate herbal mixtures and massage to apply.

When the infant begins the transition to being a young child, attention to its bowels and bladder shifts from the volume and quality of the flow to a consideration for the appropriate place for such acts. Slowly the child learns to defecate away from the household area and the village, though not necessarily away from the view of others, a consideration for modesty which develops much later. This change in concern, from the nature and quality of the substances, to the proper way to deliver oneself of them, is marked by a change in language. This is not captured in any of the dictionaries I consulted, but was often remarked upon by my informants. The polite word for faeces is *otaota*, explained to me as a pun on ripe banana meat, something Samoans find repulsive and inedible. The vernacular word is *tae* [usually pronounced kae]. *Tae* is from a class of words usually reserved for reference to animals or animal behaviour, and except as an insult, is never applied to an adult's faeces. It is also not applied to the faeces of an infant, the verb *ti'o* [to defecate] being used most often as a noun in reference to this. However, it is used even in polite conversation between members of the same sex to refer to the faeces of young children. They are learning, one mother explained, "how to shit like pigs so that then they can learn how to shit like Samoans." Slowly, during this period when defecating is moved further and further away from the village centre, the child comes to understand that his or her bowels must move, must always be flowing. However, unlike animals, their products need to be taken away from the dignified and social centre of the village and into the bush. Even so, children show little embarrassment over excretory functions. Walking in the bush, it not unusual for children to simply step off the path a foot or two and relieve themselves, while carrying on their conversation with you. A favourite game among young boys up to about the age of 10 is a competitive "who can pee further" contest in which several young boys will lift their *lavalava,* or pull their penises out of their shorts, and try to outdo each other in both distance and volume. The game reinforces, through enactment, the standard against which healthy urination is measured.

Girls begin this process of moving their excretory functions out of sight much earlier than boys, and greater caution is taken to avoid being seen. While catching young girls urinating in the bush does not cause a great deal of embarrassment, young girls learn to seek out secluded spots to urinate or defecate earlier than boys.

Moved away from the village and, relatively at least, out of sight, excretory functions finally become private ones late in childhood. The waste functions of the bowels and genitals become linked to the process of sexing bodies, which also takes place over the course of childhood, culminating in the linguistic marking of boys and girls at the period just prior to puberty [*tama tane*, boy and *tama fafine*, girl and *fa'afafine*, a biological male, but neither male nor female]. While Samoans certainly recognize the sex of their children from birth, both male and female infants and very young children are subjected to the same rules of treatment and modesty, and to the same expectations in terms of body function, until well into their childhood years. By about 4 or 5, however, the often naked boys and girls begin to be covered in some form of clothing. At the time that *tamaititi* are beginning to learn the basic rules of propriety about body waste, they are also beginning to learn genital modesty. Beyond a certain age, although there is no consensus on the limits of this age, boys and girls should no longer see each others' genitals, referred to politely from this point on as *mea sā*, or sacred things. This is the beginning of the formalization of the brother-sister relationship, a relationship of profound importance in *Fa'a Samoa* [Good 1980; Schoeffel 1979]. It is based on respect and protection of the sister by her brother, and on obedience and deference of the sister toward her brother. Its beginnings are enacted on, and with, the body, through the gradual transformation of the genitals into special things. However, genitals are not being hidden or denied, they are being located in their appropriate space. What happens, as Lacan has noted, is that in the social sexing of bodies, "... words, titles, clothes, accoutrements ... are, barring the actual *seeing* of the genitals, the 'essence' of the human 'sexed' being" [cited in MacCannell 1986:50]. Clothing, privacy, and modesty enact a new body location, signified by a deflection of attention away from the actual genitals, toward their socially charged implications. They are transformed from things to signs of and for things, that is, into social processes rather than simply socially defined objects. There is an element of disguise in the enactment of the socialized body, although it is not the fact of the disguise that is important but what the disguise points to. That is, disguise allows dangerous, ambiguous or troublesome things to be deployed in social action by serving as a buffer which neutralizes but does not eliminate them. Like euphemism, the elaboration of the body through disguise allows perilous but necessary things to exist in the social field but constrains their danger by allusion, and not deception. As Foucault and others have noted, the elaboration of discourse surrounding artifacts of social risk, in this instance the masque of dissembling diacritics through which the body is encoded in order to be decoded safely, does not eliminate the risk and may even increase it. Most importantly, it creates a grammar of risk management, if you will, which makes dangerous bodies liveable.

The function of the genitals is being divided, from solely excretory, to a combination of excretory, erotogenic and reproductive potentials. They become sex organs in both senses: organs which sex the individual and as organs used to have sex but only as potentialities. I have argued elsewhere that Samoans do not so much have genitals as they enact them, depending on the contexts in which they are deployed. Rather than bodily organs, genitals might better be characterised as embodied conditions [Drozdow-St.Christian 1992, 1993, 1994]. Childhood play that involves genital touching is not discouraged in mixed sex groups during the earliest years of childhood, but by the rough mid-point in this period [age 4 to 6], genital play among girls, or between boys and girls, is prohibited out of fear the girl's organs may be damaged. It is encouraged among boys well into adolescence, in order to strengthen the muscular aspects of their penis and testicles.

An important point about these organs needs to be stressed here. Samoans have three distinctive sexes, rather than two. That is, there are men, women and *fa'afafine*. The *fa'afafine* are genetically male in that they have penises. They use their penises in exactly the same way as males do: in heterosexual intercourse, urination, and in abiding by rules about modesty and exposure. However, the *fa'afafine* are not male, and their penises are not male sex organs. They are *fa'afafine* organs. That is, sex organs, but not ones which define the *fa'afafine* as male. My interpretation of Samoan sexes differs sharply from the discussion of "third" genders and sexes in Herdt [1994], and instead picks up on Butler's argument that sexualized biology needs to be prefigured analytically in order to understand the constructed nature of biological realities themselves [Butler 1993]. The difficulty appears to be in the way we distinguish analytically between sexes and genders, as between things and roles which follow from things. For Samoans, there is no distinction which seems to make any sense to me, since roles and the sexing things which are meant to follow from each other are actually deployed in such a way that it is the role—that is the active context—which creates the thing rather than vice versa. That means that sexing is deeply ambiguous, at least analytically. In practice, however, it remains as easy as falling off a bike for Samoans, something my dear Samoan friend Albert repeatedly told me Samoans were very good at indeed.

At the same time, unlike male and female, *fa'afafine* is a temporary sex which is abandoned later in life. This transience is important because it embodies principles of transgression and ambiguity in the embodiment of fundamental differences between individuals, something which Samoan sociality strives to disguise. The issue of genitals and gendering is important in Samoa, because these momentarily gendering roles map onto physical aspects of the body distinctive orders of meaning and experience not encompassed by the scientific classification of human bodies as male and female. As I noted in Chapter 2, the question of sexing, gender, and *fa'afafine* in Samoa is the focus of my own ongoing research. While I will restrict my comments here to boys and girls, what I say about male and female bodies can be applied equally to *fa'afafine* bodies as well, at least during childhood. Bodily praxis changes in subtle and complex ways later in life.

This shifting of excretory functions away from the centre of the village is an important aspect of learning how to embody the properties of good and proper space. In Chapter 3, I described the conceptual layout of Samoan villages, where the core of the village, most often the *malae* or sacred green, is the most dignified space. The further one moves away from the centre, the less the dignity, and the greater the danger. This slow shifting of human excretory functions into the undignified periphery of village space is an example of how intimate daily practices generate and sustain this very important distinction. In this, one can see the gradual embodiment of the world around the child in the way the child begins to engage different aspects of space with its body. The child learns early into its childhood years that what it does with its body is both determined by, and determines the nature and quality of the space in which it is moving. Space becomes an extension of his or her body, and associations of propriety, gender, dignity, and danger, become fundamental aspects of the landscape within which the child moves. The relationship between bodies in space and bodies creating space through their actions collapses into a single phenomenon in which the social nature of space, both as a material thing and as a location, or place, becomes fetishized. The complex circularity of connection between bodies and spaces in which neither creates the other, but instead taken together create some other thing, is naturalized and rendered socially invisible, and so all the more socially potent. These early moments of "toilet training" are indeed of fundamental importance, because in them the world as we can "know" it is being brought into existence.

Excretory functions, along with the emergence of the entailments surrounding sexing, are one way through which children begin their embodied transition to fuller personhood. The gustatory functions, combining appetites and the process of digestion, is another. Infants, and very young children, are fed on demand, because Samoans understand that impeding appetites, and their satisfaction, risks injuring the still developing digestive organs of young children. By age 3 or 4, children's demands for food are often ignored. While little effort is made at this point in children's lives to prevent them from finding food on their own, caregivers stop being sources of food whenever the child demands it. Even the youngest child will eat with its family at the regularly scheduled meals, although no great attention is paid to bad eating habits in the very young. Midway through the *aso fa'a tamaititi*, the childhood years, discipline begins to be applied to appetites with increasing vigour. Children learn to wait until adults have taken their portions, to eat only when told they may, and to share their food whenever asked.

Hunger and thirst are important aspects of the organic body, markers of body processes present in all human experience. People in all societies deal with these primal urges in some way. For Samoans, hunger expresses emptiness since nutrition is understood as deriving from having sufficient food in the body at all times. Faeces is not what is left after the body has removed what it needs from the food it takes in. Instead, faeces is food being pushed through the digestive system by new food, by the movement of the body at work and, as Albert put it one day, "because everything falls down sometime, Douglass." Satisfying hunger involves putting sufficient food, softened by chewing, into the body to sustain this reservoir of material for the body to use as it is needed. The formal phrase for digestion is *fa'a malō I le puta*, which combines the three senses of *malō*—to soften, fishing weir, and storage basket—and *puta*, fat. Literally, the phrase combines "to cause fat to be softened," "to catch fat in a net" and "to put fat in the basket." My informants would often refer to digestion as "carrying fat" and link the presence of fat on the body to digestion. Layers of fat are part of the stomach's normal storing function.

In infancy, because the body is still forming, it is difficult for this reserve of food to remain in place. Infants need to be fed, and overfed, in order to ensure sufficient nutrition at all times. During the early years of childhood, when children have now developed the physical ability to retain food, the habit of eating in excess has often become engrained. There is considerable tolerance during this period for immoderate, and on demand eating by children. Slowly, however, children learn about the properties of food and its relationship to their bodies, and it is during this period that they also learn restraint. However, this should not be mistaken for something as simple as postponement of gratification. It is tied to biology, on the one hand, and to increasing social awareness on the other. Children come to understand that hunger is not an alarm, or a signal of distress. Instead, hunger tells them they will need to eat again, not simply that they need to eat now. The body holds food, it does not absorb it, and hunger simply indicates that the body will soon need to be refilled. The social awareness, written out in the way they deal with hunger, relates to an understanding of the nature of social support among Samoans. "There is always food here because everyone helps everyone, so no one can starve," I was told, "but children do not know this, not for a long time. Children think about food like something that might go away, might never be there. Only later do they know there is always food." In learning to postpone the satisfaction of hunger, children are learning, with their bodies, core principles of Samoan sociality, in particular the value of sharing and mutual support. They are learning their bodies need food, the language by which their body reminds them they need food, and also that there is always food. Hunger, they learn, is a reminder of the basic character of community concern, support, and sharing.

One sees this series of lessons most poignantly in the practice of auto-constipation, especially among middle aged [5 to 7 years] children of very poor families. I did not fully understand the biology of digestion as storage until a mother told me about problems she had had with her two sons when they were about 5 or 6 years old. Because of serious disputes within their 'āiga, and the loss of the household's only cash job, the family had experienced a long period when food was scarce. During this time, both her sons became very ill, and when examined by a fofō [Samoan healer], it was revealed that they had intentionally not had bowel movements in several days, in order to prevent what food remained in their bodies from being evacuated. A kind of community based family counselling, in which the two boys were reassured by all members of their village that they would always have enough food, along with massage and a purgative, were needed to correct the boys' physical problem, and to help them learn these fundamental body lessons.

Weight loss and weight gain follow closely monitored patterns in young children. After passing through the first year of life, a child is expected to begin to lose weight such that by age 6 or so, Samoan children are often quite small and wiry. Average weight of young children, as well as average rates of growth beyond infancy, are well below the median for such averages found among American children [Bindon and Zansky 1986:227]. Parents explain this as the result of children's need to run about and to be constantly on the move. "Children," I was told "have not learned to be still [manava, which is also "to breathe"], because they still do not know everything about the village and their family" and so "they become small because they are always running. They will learn to be still later."[2]

This pattern of weight loss is enforced through surveillance and comment on the state of children's weight. A fat 6-year-old child is the object of either scorn or concern, is called le puta [the noun form of fat], and his parents and caregivers are often queried by other family and village members. Is the child sick, they will ask, or is he arrogant, having adopted an

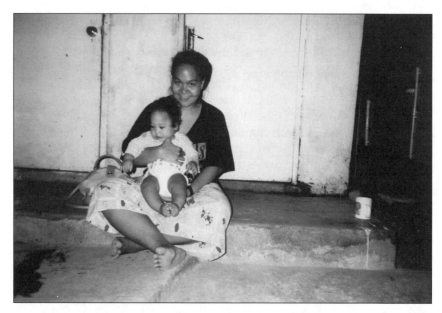

Figure 5.1 A healthy six-month-old infant
[*tamameamea*] is fat, alert, curious and active.

adult body style prematurely, or is he not learning the proper manner of
Samoan children, that is, learning restraint and orderly eating? Not only
adults reinforce this concern. The most common form of name calling
among children refers to obesity. Children's insults are an interesting source
of information on the acquisition of cultural values and ideas about the
world. While I did not collect data on this area of children's interactions
systematically, I did note a pattern to children's insults and criticisms of
other children, which focusses almost exclusively on the body. Along with
obesity, children also comment critically on the cleanliness of their peers,
and on their lack of strength.

Gradually this process of weight loss is reversed, so that by the beginning of the *tama* or young person phase of their development [about 12 to
13 years], boys and girls begin to put weight back on [Bindon and Zan-
sky:244-247]. This begins earlier for girls than boys, explained by girls'
greater need for additional mass to allow for the proper formation of the
breasts. In both girls and boys, this weight gain is understood as part of their
transformation into reproductive adults, fat acting as a buffering and warming protection for the internal organs, or the internal spaces, where reproductive substances are formed, stored and, in the *fa'aautagata*, combined in the foetus. This pattern of weight gain and loss is illustrated in
the photographs on the next several pages.

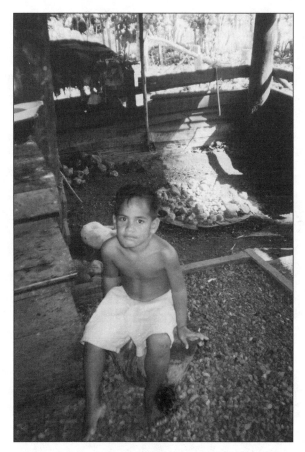

Figure 5.2 By four years old, Samoan children have lost their infant fat, and rate of growth has slowed.

It closely parallels increases in dignity and status as Samoans mature and grow older. Adolescent weight gain is gendered, girls gaining more weight than boys, but by the time of their late twenties and early thirties, both men and women begin to gain weight in comparable amounts. By their mid to late 50's, both men and women have average weights of close to 200 pounds [Pawson 1986:262]. This weight gain is likely a result of the connection between status over the life course, and eating practices. Samoans are remarkable eaters. They can consume monumental amounts of food everyday. This food is heavy in starches, such as taro and rice, and also has a high fat content because so many dishes are prepared using beef tallow. At the same time, as a person matures into their 40's, they are ex-

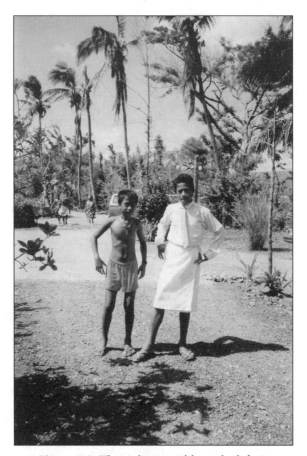

Figure 5.3 The eight year old, on the left, is typical of older Samoan children [*tamaititi*] in being thin and wiry. His twelve-year-old brother, in white, has begun the transition to adolescence and is beginning to gain weight once again.

pected to do less and less physical labour. The normative status which attaches to maturity means that middle-aged Samoans supervise manual labour, rather than participate directly in it. A combination of an increasingly sedentary lifestyle and a high fat, high carbohydrate diet, results in mid-life obesity in almost all Samoans. This is more an intuitive observation, than a nutritional one. Hanna, Pelletier and Brown note that "attemps to link daily food intake to obesity...have not been successful [1986:295]. Samoan's own perception of the material causes of weight

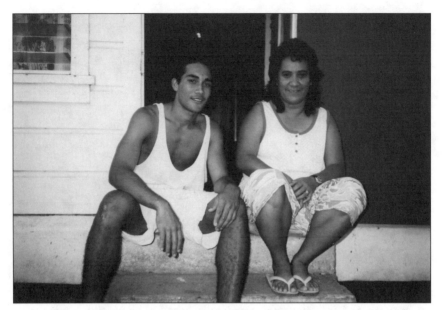

Figure 5.4 A young man and woman in their early twenties. Young women begin the process of weight gain earlier than young men.

gain are, as one man put it, "the respect a person should have when he is a mature and important man."

While Pawson's data on the morphology of adult Samoans, noted above, does not control for titled or untitled status, there appears to be a relationship between weight, and holding a *matai* title. However, it is a relationship of relative massiveness. That is to say, *matai* were, from my subjective observations, usually the largest men in a village. However, almost all men in the villages I worked in were very large by their early 50's. Adult sons of *matai* are also, subjectively at least, larger than their peers, a subject which my informants often commented on. Many felt that the sons of *matai* were too arrogant and immodest, "acting like they are princes, and not just our brothers." Some of the *matai's* sons, themselves, were aware of this disparity, commenting on how lower status men should be small because, in one man's words, "they are the smallest of all the people in *Fa'a Samoa*." Relative weight has become a marker of class distinction for some Samoans. However, while titled and untitled status does not currently define a fixed class for most Samoans, the question of class in Samoa is changing. The extension of suffrage to all adult Samoans, in 1989, has generated a conflict between *matai*, and the untitled members of their *'āiga*. A small, but vocal, group of *matai* are agitating for a repeal of the legislative amendments which granted universal suffrage, on the grounds that

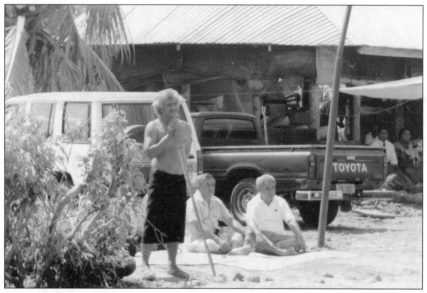

Figure 5.5 A *tulafale matai*, speaking on behalf of his *ali'i*, seated, in the white shirt. The *tulafale* is around 45 years old while the *ali'i* was 66 at the time of this photograph. Note the differences in size of the two men, reflecting different stages in the life course.

only *matai* have the moral and cultural authority to enact political decisions. This authority does not extend to imposing decisions on their untitled family members, since political decision-making remains a process of consensus among all '*āiga* members. However, the dispute over suffrage has planted some very tentative seeds of fixed distinction into this relationship between consensus and the authority to act, and many Samoans are expressing an increasing disatisfaction with what they see as an increased arrogance on the part of *matai* as a group, using such markers are body size to site this dissatisfaction. The possibility exists that physical markers of an emergent class status may become more important in the future, as this controversy over suffrage and authority continues. While detailed discussion of the changes in the relations of authority and power in Samoa is beyond the scope of this text, it is useful to note that the body may play a key role in the way these changes develop over the next several years.[3]

I could see no observable difference in relative size among wives of high status, and of lower status husbands. Samoan's expect all adults to grow in weight throughout their lives, and enquire after a person's health if they feel they are too thin, or too fat for their age. Later in life, both men and women lose weight, which was explained as the slow degradation of the body's ability to draw energy and strength from food.

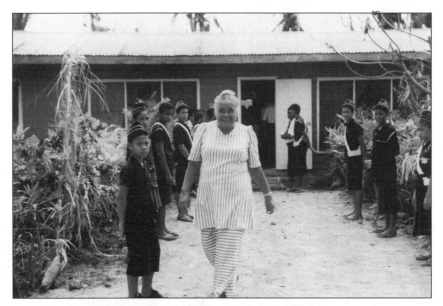

Figure 5.6 The 59-year-old wife of an important *matai*, she is typical in weight and stature of Samoan women at this age.

Sexing is implicated in other changes in the gustatory functions, that is, in the practices surrounding nutrition and eating. This area of cultural enactment has been described by Kahn [1986], and Meigs [1983], for two societies in New Guinea, addressing issues of gender, power, and spirituality in practices surrounding the growing, preparation, and consumption of food. However, Meigs, for example, locates food, both in its meanings and its practices, at the heart of an imperfect recollection of traditional culture among the Hua, arguing that it is "an ideology as it is remembered…by a group whose culture is now in decline" [1983:xv]. In contrast, I am arguing that the relationships between eating, food, and the good and proper body, are indivisible particles of a vibrant and ongoing enactment of tradition and culture in Samoa.[4]

Girls and boys have similar capacities and needs for food. However, eating habits begin to diverge during the middle period of the *aso fa'a tamaititi*. Gradually girls learn to chew their food more thoroughly than boys, because girls' nutrition is based on the ability of food material to pass into the blood, while boys' involves food material being taken up in the denser tissue of muscle and bone. At the same time, girls learn to allow boys to eat first when they are fed together, while boys learn to leave the best portions of dishes for their sisters to eat. Boys get more while girls get better. In part, this is an expression of the complex relationship of re-

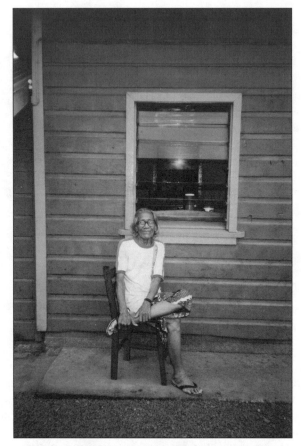

Figure 5.7 A 78-year-old woman, once a robust 200 pounds. This photograph was taken several months before her death from "old age."

spect and deference which exists between brothers and sisters, but in part it is an expression of an emerging sense of a gendered biology as well. Girls require finer food for their blood, which is a finer substance, but boys require greater bulk because boys move more, more quickly, and for longer periods of time than girls. This is not simply a matter of different roles, however. Girls have slower, though not weaker, muscles than boys because of the dominance of blood in their physical makeup. Boys on the other hand have faster moving muscles, though again, not necessarily stronger muscles than girls. In this division of food, and in acts of deference and the orderly sharing of food, children are engaging in an embodiment of meanings about how bodies work and how sexed bodies work differently.

At the same time that children are learning the biological distinctions between boys and girls, and their relationship to food, digestion, and genitals, they are also beginning to learn about food as an embodiment of principles of status and authority.[5] Food, whether traditional or imported foodstuffs, is ranked not only in reference to its nutritive value, but also by colour [white and not-white], the manner in which it is cooked [boiled, fried, or roasted in the *umu* (earth oven)], and by rules about who may, or at least should, eat this particular food. During infancy and the earliest period of the *aso fa'a tamaititi*, children are served the highest status food available, white and boiled food. This most often takes the form of rice, the status of which is enhanced by the fact it must be bought with cash, and is considered a valuable imported *palagi* or European food. As a child progresses through its childhood years, a gradual shift in diet occurs. While sustaining the white and imported association all the way through to adulthood in the use of *saimin*, packaged dried noodle soups imported from China and Japan, children also begin to eat a wider range of foods, and to learn the status associations between kinds of food and the parts of foodstuffs. For example, boiled food such as bananas and taro, which are ideally prepared only by men, are among the highest status everyday foodstuffs in the Samoan diet. By their middle childhood years [age 4 to 6], children are fed these foods less and less often, although they are encouraged to ask for them. This combination of encouraging requests, and consistently refusing them, teaches the child the importance of these status associations. Other food is reserved exclusively for adults. *Palusami*, a pudding of coconut cream baked in young taro leaves, is almost never eaten by children, or even untitled adults, so precious are the leaves in which the pudding is cooked. Likewise, fish is rarely served to children, being defined almost exclusively as adult food. On special occasions, and these are indeed quite rare, children will be given servings of *pisupo*, tinned corned beef. This is treated as a special gift, and the child is warned to take its small portion and no more, because *pisupo* is not food for children. Finally, portions of food, such as the parts of a roasted pig, or the parts of a fish, are associated with particular statuses. The head of the fish, along with the relatively meatless rib portion of the pig, are defined as the *matai*'s portion. Very young children will often ask for servings from these portions, usually from their titled grandfather or uncle. Depending on the mood of the *matai*, he may indulge the child with a scrap of skin or fat, but in every instance I witnessed, the *matai* would first explain that this was *matai* food, and that the child should not ask for such things. During the hundreds of meals in which I took part, I never once saw a child over the age of 5 or 6 even ask for a serving of the *matai*'s portion. When I questioned older children and young adults about the distribution of food at meals, they were unanimous in their attitude that it would be extremely insulting and ignorant for anyone except a *matai* to accept (let alone ask for), any part of these portions of the animals. I received several explanations for the associations between parts of the roasted pig, for example, and the people expected to eat them. The guest portion of a roasted pig is the ham, the meatiest and most substantial portion of the animal and expresses generosity and respect to visitors. The *matai's* portion, the ribs and back, express several different associations. The ribs are "like the house posts where the *matai* sit in meetings and remind us of this." The ribs also encompass the *manava* of the pig, the sacred core to the body, and by the *matai* eating the rib portion "we learn about how the *matai* is the core of our family and our village."

Embedded in this ranking and classification of foods are complex rules of order, authority and status, something noted by others working in Samoa, in particular Mageo [1989b], where she uses a detailed symbolic analysis of a Samoan song to link questions of eating and speaking behaviour in Samoa, to the process through which children and adults learn about delinquency and obedience. While my focus here is on how eating behaviour, and ideas about food, affects the experience of the body, this dimension of socialization through the body is worth noting. At the same time, I am focusing solely on regular meals which then misses the equally compelling and complex rules and embodying practices surrounding who can eat, where they are allowed to eat, and how place determines in many instances what can be eaten. There is, for example, a distinction between personal or individual acts of eating and those which occur collectively, and the rules regarding eating in public, which is ideally prohibited. I recall an ice cream outlet in Apia, not particularly large but always packed with people, sardine like, eating their rapidly melting cones. Pushed onto the sidewalk by the crush, people would attempt to step back into the shops opening rather than stand in some more exposed and public space like the roadway. This is interesting because the shop front was actually completely open to the street but it was in a metaphorical sense, and so in an embodied one, not quite a public space. In contrast, food distributed to people "watching" a funeral, that is, people on the periphery not taking direct part in the funerals processes, is often as not eaten on the roadside or by groups of people walking back along the road from the village in which the funeral was taking place. These groups of "observers" included both *tulafale* and *ali'i* not directly or indirectly involved in the funeral proceedings, breaching a fundamental prohibition against *matai* eating in some space defined as public. Eating alone in private, and especially eating alone and in public, has connotations of greed, of standing out or above others. But eating in public as part of a group, that is in a commu-

nal meal even if a moving and very public one, does not carry these connotations at all. The body is engaged here in a remarkable set of maneu-
vers through which public and private, social and anti-social, sharing and
obligation, to name a few, a enacted by being engaged. All of these things
are played out in those more formal meals, and I will return shortly to the
most special all meals in Samoa, the Sunday mid-day meal, but I want to
at least acknowledge that eating is more than just family dinners.

The child, as he or she becomes more and more a full participant in
mealtimes, rather than something to be fed, learns these rules literally on
the end of its fork, or the tips of its greasy fingers. The association between
food and the good and proper order of status and authority cannot be
avoided, even in something so apparently mundane as eating an evening
meal. Children are learning and practicing principles of strength, authority, dignity and modesty, not only in the way they learn to endure hunger
by revising its meaning into something positive rather than something
alarming, but in the way they begin to relate kinds of food to the needs
of the body's growth and development as a strong and proper body. They
learn the differences in strengths between the strength of the *matai* expressed in his repose and humility, and the strength of the young men able
to carry loads of coconuts over several miles without complaint. They are
learning about the importance of steadiness and endurance as components
of the Samoan model of strength, lessons reinforced by their craving for food
appropriate to generating strength. The meaning of the body, and the way
the body is made meaningful, becomes attached, inexorably, to the meaning of food and the practices of eating. Eating taro enacts strength, while
a *matai* eating the head of a fish embodies the power and authority attached to his status.

Mealtime enacts another form of body learning, that involving movement and posture. Very young children are fed with the rest of the family,
but they sit to the side, and slightly behind the parent or caregiver who is
feeding them. Food is passed to them, either on a plate or leaf, or cut into
chewable single mouthfuls. Behind their feeder, the child is often rambunctious, noisy and fidgety. Little attention is paid to this movement and
noise, unless it becomes so disturbing as to interrupt some important family conversation.

By the time the child reaches the age of about 4, however, he or she begins to take a place in the family circle, sitting beside a parent or caregiver,
and taking their own portions of food from the plates of goods delivered
by older children. They are chastised if they are noisy, or move about too
much, and they now begin to have their posture corrected. All Samoans,
when sitting on the ground, sit with their legs crossed under their torso. To
sit with your legs extended, or oriented in any other way, is considered
rude because, in traditional dress, to sit any other way makes exposure of

the genitals or buttocks a very real possibility. Even in shorts or trousers, children by about age 4 are being taught to sit cross legged, that is, to "sit like a human being and not a dog." One man scolded his married daughter for not yet teaching her 6-year-old daughter how to sit properly and on several occasions both the mother and daughter were ordered to leave the family meal, and take their dinner "with the dogs down by the river." Rudeness is not the only consideration however. The cross legged posture also restricts movement. It must be entered into, and extricated from, slowly. Once sitting, apart from waving your arms about, movement is severely circumscribed. This closing in of the body into an attitude of stillness is an aspect of embodiment which children learn in several ways, but it is in the family circle at mealtime that they receive the closest and most detailed lesson. During mealtime the person eating becomes like the still heart of the village, around which activity circulates, but does not intrude. In this posture, the child is learning a lesson about doing and being still in which the conceptual landscape of the village is embodied in postural language.

At the same time, the complex moral geography of the meal with its ordering of who eats, when, and what sorts of food, reinforces a different sort of embodied posture in which the body deployed in this morally charged space of eating is re-inforcing, and enforcing, an orderly embodiment of propriety and space. You will recall that the village is oriented spatially from its still, and sacred, centre outward to the darkness of the asocial, and even potentially anti-social space of the plantation and the wild. In parallel, the household itself mimics this spatial deployment with the centre of the *fale* standing for the *malae*, and in circles of decreasing sociality and dignity, radiating outward to the space where the household engages the dangers of the wild. The family at a meal is yet another instance of the place of this morally ordered space in which the web of extensive connection which is the *'āiga* as a whole is centred in the contrived moral stillness of the meal, as the immediate family — an immediate family whose makeup is driven by the days context of visits and obligations, however — becomes like the *malae* itself, a still and sacred embodied enactment of the flow of action and responsibility in Samoan sociality. As the child joins this circle of duty and conviviality, learns to sit cross legged and await her portion, to know what portion is indeed hers, and to come to understand and participate in the process of sharing and support which the meal expresses, she is making a morally centred physical world with her hands and teeth and stomach. The meal does not simply reinforce the orderliness of moral embodiment, it is a fundamental, and fundamentally regulated creation of that orderliness.

This lesson of proper bodies, properly still in some centre of social activity, is not only learned during meals. In their everyday play, they also learn about the appropriate meaning of different forms of space. Very young children play around their household compound, and on the *malae* or public area of the village. Play is not sexed until very late in a child's development, when girls learn to refrain from extremely rowdy play, and boys beginning pursuing such often violent and intense games as rugby. Throughout childhood, and sometimes up into the early teens, but prior to the development of secondary sexual characteristics, children play together irrespective of sex, the only caution being to keep the genitals covered.

Gradually, however, children learn to restrain the noise and commotion of their play in the central areas of the village, and to reserve rowdiness for the periphery. It is not unusual to see children returning from school chase each other, laughing and calling loudly as they come along the village road. As they approach the *malae*, or its equivalent, they become quieter, and move more and more slowly, not stopping their game, but restraining it, only to explode into laughter and running as they move away from the *malae* and into the household area. Whether it is the nature of the space that restrains their bodies, or their embodiment itself which transforms the space as they move into and through it is a moot point. I have been stressing that the two can never be analytically separated into cause and effect. Body and space become each other and create each other, whether in the slow walk of the children through the *malae,* or the soft speech of women walking at night, speech which erupts into laughter as they move deeper into the periphery of the village.

Hunger, bowel movements and children's games, posture and the social meanings of food: each of these, and the other things the body is engaged in, form the complex web of practices I am defining here as embodiment. Each is both an effect of the body, and has an effect on the body. Watching 4-year-old Heston play around the windows of my house in the late afternoon sun—watching him take several stones and roll them around each other, singing softly to himself, then suddenly stand and look around before dashing behind a bush to pee against the stoop, I was watching what was little more than a charming scene, during the first months I spent in Samoa. After I left Samoa, the full and rich analytic complexity of that tiny scene became clear to me. In those early stages I was doing what Samoan parents do during those first crucial months of an infant's life. I was recognizing the body in front of me, Heston's tiny body, as some object worth noting. I was recognizing it, but I was not understanding it. I was not seeing what Heston himself was doing as he created and navigated the meanings and implications of his presence as a body in the world.

The process of attention, then, has shifted from the simple act of someone observing a thing, such as parents watching their infants bowels, and drawing meaning from it, to a more subtle process of attention, in which the observed thing, the child, is attending to its own being and, by doing so, making itself, and the world meaningful and observable.

Attention has shifted in other ways as well, from the ego-object focus of the infant on its own body alone, to a wider focus on the relationships between things in the social field. The child's body is no longer the centre, but is, instead, a component in the complex machinery of connected things. The meaningful body of the infant, whose features and qualities were measured and standardized, becomes, in the process of learning to be a body, a shifting thing requiring constant attention, vigilance, and re-interpretation. Faeces, for example, is necessary and good. It is evidence of a good and proper body. At the same time it is being moved further and further away from the visual core of the village into the asocial and *lēaga* space of the bush. Strength, that ability to run long and hard, which is expressed in childhood play with all its rowdiness and noise, is also improper, immodest, and inappropriate depending on the space body is in. Genitals, once solely the site of bodily needs, or simple pleasure and games, remain so, but with an additional mapping of other genitals with other obligations, prohibitions, and consequences. Hunger, that gross appetite for satisfaction which is never denied or prohibited, has become encompassed by considerations of status, propriety, and power, as well as trust, obligation and restraint.

What I have been describing here is, perhaps, the least special, and also the least observed aspect of being in the world. It is transparent, but its transparency is part of its effect. Behind the self evident presence of Heston deciding where to urinate, the complicated web of attention and action which is the core of embodiment is carried out both in, and on, the world.

Heston lay across my bed, asleep in the deepening darkness of a very rainy night, just hours before Cyclone Val struck the north-west coast of the island of Upolu. We had been preparing for the cyclone for three days, tying hoardings around the *fale* which sits behind my *palagi* bungalow and trying to herd together the family's pigs into a sheltered area which we hope will remain above the rising flood waters of the blocked Gasegase Stream. From somewhere in the distance I hear a woman calling someone's name, but with the tricks of the wind, and the constant battering of the rain against my tin roof, I can't quite make out who she is calling. I draw back the canvas covering we had secured earlier that day on the windows along the front of my house, and shine my flashlight through the rain, trying to pick out where I think the voice is coming from. As I do, Heston wakes up and crawls across the bed, reaching over, and pulling himself up onto my back, so he can see what I am doing.

"Aiku?" he asks.

"Sione. I think she is calling Tagilima."

"Sione not aiku."

"No, stinky Heston is aiku."

"You aiku, Doug. You stinky too, stinky *palagi* aiku with big feet."

"And a big mouth that is going to eat you up if you don't get off my back and go back to sleep."

"No eat Heston, Heston too little."

"I like little things, they're easier to chew."

"I eat big things, big taro and big pig, and then Heston eats you, Doug, eats you because you are too small, you eat lady food, you eat like a girl, only small things like a girl. Heston gets big and stinky from taro and pua'a, and eats the little soft girl Doug."

I was just a soft, stinky, girlish, *palagi*, with big feet. Heston, with his bad jokes, constant questions, and his embodied Samoan common sense, knew this. He was a 4-year-old child, trying to make a joke with a man ten times his age, in a language, and in a universe of concepts and anticipations, that he understood because he enacted them everyday. At the time I thought of Heston as a precocious and charming child. It was only later, on reflection, that I recognized the complex accomplishment Heston enacted with his silly, embodying jokes.

The central issue I have raised in this chapter, is that ultimately and finally, the body cannot be said to exist at all, until it is attended to. Deciphering the how, and the what, of attention, is one route into the generation of a comprehensive model of embodiment: that is, a model of those practices and experiences, which Heston does without thinking, and with aplomb, as he moves through his childhood, enacting attention on his body, and on the world.

With 4-year-old Heston making sense of the world in mind, I want to turn, in the next chapter, to issues of the orderly deployment of disciplined bodies, in order to explore the process of embodiment at several different points in its continuous enactment. Learning a proper body, as an act of being a body in the world, is only one aspect of this process. It is the ground on which all other action is made possible, and I want to look at some other kinds of enacted bodies that flow from this primary site of attention.

Chapter 6

The Statutory Body:
Discipline and Control

Discipline, pleasure, and obligation cannot be disentangled from the deployment of social bodies in Samoa. The implications of embodiment are always, whatever the mundaneness of the action, a connection between the body, and the wider processes of authority and obedience. At the same time, the complexity of each individual Samoan's network of relationships of obligation, and the different levels of dignity and restriction which apply to kinds of space, mean there is ample room for transgression and manipulation. In the acts of pleasure and cooperation, dignity, discipline and responsibility are performed both on and through the body. In this section, I will describe some of the more formal locations and practices in which constrained and disciplined bodies are enacted in Samoa. I will deal in turn with the ceremonial deployments of the 'ava [kava — piper methysticum] preparation and distribution ceremony, tattooing and circumcision, and punishment and apology, exploring the link between discipline and the embodiment of proper space.

Discipline in the mundane sense of punishing wrongdoing or error is, to be blunt, brutal and immediate in Samoa. In infancy and earliest childhood, there is little if any discipline, rarely going beyond whispered admonitions of 'aua or soia, both words generally used in speaking to animals, and both translating as "stop that." In the early years of childhood, caregivers will begin using two different admonitions. The first, uma, which means enough, this is finished, entails a different mode of control which is about sufficiency and excess, and the line between them. "Play loudly, for a while," it says, "but this is the limit. No more, at least not for now." The other, the exhortation "oo-ee," for which there is no written equivalent, is a marker of shame. To have someone call "oo-ee" in respect of something you are doing is to be told what you are doing is shameful and, with uma, "oo-ee" becomes the most common register for indicating displeasure to children aged around 5 or so [Ochs 1988:153-155]. In later years, the use of "oo-ee" directed at an adult is considered a way of telling the miscreant to stop behaving like a child.

At the same time that social responsibility is being encoded in expressions of displeasure, physical discipline becomes harsher and more violent. It is not unusual for children, aged 6 and older, to be severely beaten. The intensity of these beatings increases with age. By adolescence discipline can be as serious as hanging by an incensed parent.

Discipline is tied to what a person should know, that is, what rules a person should be aware of. "When a baby shits on the *malae* it is stupid, like a pig, but when a boy shits on the *malae*, it is *lēaga* and he should be beaten, he should be reminded and he should learn." Discipline is *pulega*, the application of appropriate authority and power. *Pulega* is not power imposed, but authority anticipated, and, as Shore [1982:158-160] has noted as well, punishment is almost universally acknowledged as good and proper, most specifically by those being punished. Punishment is also finite. A punished person is almost immediately reintegrated into his or her family and community following a beating or other punishment. The act of punishment, *fa'a sala*, is the path from a mistake, the ending of an error, and the direction an offender takes back toward communal participation. The physical act of punishment does not avenge the offense, it reminds the offender of the way out of the mistake and back into complete and responsible sociality. Samoan justice, *amiotonu*, is an agreement on proper behaviour, and not an abstract principle of right. As well, it is restorative and not retributive [Shore 1982:116-117].

I want to make clear, however, that compliance in Samoa is, at least in part, a function of fear about injury and pain. This makes the body a primary site in calculating the risks of disobedience as well as a primary site in restoring propriety and sustaining authority. The atmosphere of social control in Samoa is one in which real violent penalty is a constant which needs to be accounted for in all action.

Coupled with this awareness of the potential for violent penalty is a different recognition, that wrongdoing is not just about individual offenders. A murderer or a thief or a rapist, in their acts, implicates their entire family, sometimes drawing everyone in their *'āiga potopoto*, [the largest form of the extended family], into the process of punishment. Blame is distributed through the network of relations a person has, and restitution, including sometimes the imposition of violent punishment, is extensive rather than intensive. The entire *'āiga* may be punished for one person's bad actions. In accepting punishment, everyone including the actual miscreant, is participating in a process where discipline is applied to relationships as much as it is applied to individuals. As such, the ground on which bodies are disciplined and punished must not be seen as populated by finite, isolated bodies. It is a collectivity of multiple bodies, jointly responsible to each other, and to the community as a whole.

Making Correct Bodies: The Fono and the 'Ava Ceremony

Formal bodies in Samoa are most often those bodies, marked by rank, engaged in the special activities which attach to their rank. Duranti [1992], for example, describes how the welcoming speeches of *matai* at important *fono* [meetings of *matai*] are part of a process which acknowledges the status which defines their bodies as legitimate sites of important village decisions and actions, while Schoeffel [1979] discusses how the Women's Health Committee, and the Samoa mother's organization, engage female bodies in constituting the formal power of female status through rituals of leadership and deference. I want to consider two aspects of the formal embodiment of space in Samoa: the ceremonial distribution of *'ava* [piper methysticum] at meetings of *matai*, and the seating of kinds of bodies in these meetings.

The formal *'ava* preparation and drinking ceremony occurs as the opening event of all major *fono*. In it, *'ava* is prepared and ceremonially distributed to the attending *matai* following a strict set of rules of performance and status. It is a solemn and quiet moment in what are often boisterous and rancorous meetings. Through it both the *aga* [social appropriateness], and the *sā* [sacredness], of the meeting are constituted in the disciplined deployment of particular kinds of bodies in the meeting house.

The *'ava* ceremony may come either before or after the ceremonial greetings which establish the preliminary ordering of status of the participants, but there is no agreement among *matai* I spoke with as to the proper orders of business. Of all the formal *fono* I witnessed as an observer, the ceremony took place after the ceremonial greetings, and the assignment of seating positions to the attending *matai*. An older and very senior *matai* explained that "once they are seated where they must be seated, then it is time to tell them this is an important day and they should behave with importance toward it." The ordering of seating in the *fono* is a map of status and rank, as illustrated in Figure 6.1.

The layout of the *fono* is oriented to the front/back distinction I described in Chapter 3, in relation to village layout and the meanings spaces in household compounds and in houses themselves. The designations *atualuma* [to be in front], *pepe* [sides of a house], and *matuātala* [centre posts], are points on a compass of status. Seating around, and within, these areas of the house, are indications of relative rank between participants, although Shore notes that while

> status distinctions suggest a clear binary opposition, those of
> rank are appropriately graduated allowing for the expression

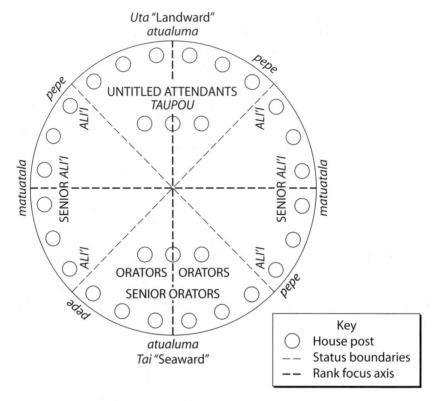

Figure 6.1 Map of Rank Locations in a Samoan *fono* [Shore 1982:80]

of subtle and gradual rank distinctions. While such a scheme theoretically permits a precise indication of rank, the tendency is for ranking distinctions to be left relatively ambiguous, with the extremes of centre posts and no post as the only clear indices of rank. This tendency suggests the reluctance of Samoans to be explicit or rigid about ranking in any but a very general way [1982:80].

Location in the *fono* is negotiated, and occasionally argued over. It shifts according to the nature of the meeting, or the presence of different *matai* whose relationships among themselves require a different orientation in ranked space.

The *ali'i*, the focal point of rank and status in an *'āiga*, are located around the central house posts, with the *tulafale* arrayed at the front of the house. Behind them sit the lower ranking *tulafale matai* and other quests. In front of them sit the ceremonial *'ava* attendants. This orientation suggests to many Samoans a form of body, where the *tulafale* are the voice of the body, the *ali'i* the head embodying the authority to act, and the attendants and lower ranking *matai* the arms and legs and digestive system, the parts of the body which sustain the rest.[1]

The ceremony begins with a silent and seductive dance by the *taupou*, the ceremonial virgin, who is most often the daughter of the most important *matai* attending the *fono*. This dance is described as a way of arousing the communal attention of the *fono* by focussing on the sensual beauty of the virgin, a figure in *Fa'a Samoa* of considerable importance [see, for example, Mageo 1998]. The attendants seated behind her, a group of untitled young men from the many villages represented in the *fono*, hold the *'ava* roots which have been brought by the various *matai*, sometimes singing softly, or quietly beating on small drums.

When the dance finishes, the *taupou* sits crosslegged in front of a large wooden *'ava* bowl and is handed portions of root which have been chewed by the attendants behind her. She takes these portions and raises them above her head, the traditional gesture acknowledging receipt of a gift, indicating that the receiver of a gift is literally under the obligation of the gift, and at the same time, not worthy of the gift received. Once the quality of the gift is acknowledged, and there is often considerable dispute over the size of the roots each *matai* has brought, she places the portions in the *'ava* bowl and, mixing them with water, begins to process the chewed root by straining it through bundles of coconut fibre until, after repeated straining and squeezing, and the addition of several more portions of chewed root, the drink is considered ready to be distributed.

The *taupou* takes the first cup of *'ava* to the ranking *tulafale*, who examines and tastes it. He either approves it, or returns it for additional portions to be added or for it to be better strained. If the drink is deemed acceptable, a long process of calling out the cup names of attending *matai*, which names are included in the formal genealogies of *matai* [*fa'alupega*], begins. As each name is called, the *taupou* takes a cup of the drink to the named *matai*, who drinks it, and exhorts the crowd with a cry of "*manuia leilei*," roughly translating as excellent health. This process proceeds through the entire assembly of *matai*. The order of distribution establishes the ranking pattern appropriate to the particular *fono* such that "an implicit weighting or ranking of 'voices' is clarified in the order of service…thus…fine-tun[ing] the decision making process" of the meeting [Shore 1982:303 n1].

The ceremony is usually, but not necessarily, repeated at the end of each sequence of speeches by *matai*, and the order of distribution may change significantly between one ceremony and the next, in the course of a single meeting. A major difference is that in later ceremonies, the *taupou* is usually replaced by one of the untitled male attendants who, by serving as the *'ava* preparer, is at least momentarily defined as a virgin.

In this ordering of bodies in the *fono*, several axes of embodiment coincide. The first relates bodies as statussed objects to the status map of social space, the seating of the *fono* a physical manifestation of rank and power in which the arrangement of the bodies literally arranges space in terms of embodied power. The process of seating the *matai* enacts status through the siting of the bodies in the *fono* house. In this way, both the ranked ordering of space, and the status entailments of the bodies of the *matai*, are created simultaneously.

At the same time a second axis of embodiment is enacted in the relationship between the seating of the *matai* and the *'ava* servers on the front/back locus. This enforces a distinction between action and stillness, the servers movement marking the *saofa'i* [the right to sit and talk] of the *matai*, and creating the code of disciplined action and immobility which attaches to good and proper bodies.

Simultaneous with this embodying of front as formal and still, and back as active and labouring, the array of server and served are mutually necessary, since the *fono* cannot legitimately function unless the untitled facilitate the exchange and consumption of *'ava*. This enacts in and through the bodies deployed in the *fono* house the mutuality of authority and compliance which is the core of Samoan power.

Finally, the performance of the *taupou* or the male "ceremonial" virgin, engages the embodying order of kinds of sexual and gendered bodies. The sensuality of the *taupou's* dance, the grace of the "virgin" boy, and the obeisance of the act of serving the *'ava* to the attending *matai*, becomes an instance of sexual tension, in which sexual bodies collude in a representation and enactment of the virtues of both constraint and eroticism. The ritual of service, like the ritual of seating the *matai* in appropriate spaces, disciplines the several bodies of the Samoan social field into the orderliness of a ranked and circumscribed world, by incorporating those bodies many sides and features. The *'ava* ceremony, and the *fono* it constitutes and permits, are formal sites of bodies being experienced through constituted in the multiple orders of meaning within which bodies act, are enacted, and are acted upon in Samoan society.

Creating Disciplined Bodies: Tattooing and Circumcision

The bodies deployed in the *fono* are public bodies enacting the public geographies of embodied order. There are also private, individualized sites of embodied order. For women, these sites include pregnancy and birth, which I discussed briefly in Chapter 4. For men, they include the connected practices of circumcision and tattooing, as well as the ritually secret practices surrounding their bodies when they are installed as a titled person. I will deal only with circumcision and male tattooing, here, but will touch on some of the aspects of masquerade in the investiture of chiefs in my conclusions.

Tattooing is a site at which discipline and the body are connected in social practice. My discussion of tattooing, tattoo designs, and tattoo interpretation is based on my own interviews with tattooists and their subjects, observations of tattoos being done and the comprehensive catalog of tattoo designs in Forsyth [1983]. However, while Forsyth is interested in cataloguing the semantics of tattoo design, I am interested in its grammar as an act of embodiment. As well, I focus on male tattoos, about which I have the most first-hand information. Female tattoos, from my limited discussions with tattooed women, appear to be about marking status moreso than they are about marking service and obligation. As such, most women I met with tattoos had taken the tattoo as a sign of their position as the wife of a ranking chief. As you will see, this is significantly different from the objective of male body marking, at least today.

The traditional male tattoo in Samoa is a dense pattern of closely drawn designs which cover the body from the midriff to the knees. All parts of the body between these limits are tattooed, except the penis and scrotum. Pubic hair is shaved, however, and the tattoo designs in some cases continue right up to the base of the penis itself. The designs included in these full body tattoos, which when completed look like a very tight fitting pair of shorts, are meaningful, but their associations in a given tattoo are more often aesthetic than narrative.[2] The tattooist chooses designs based on which he feels would best suit the shape and size of the body of his subject. There is a tradition of certain designs which symbolize or stand for, generically, fish or kinds of birds or types of waves, being associated with particular 'āiga, but there is no formal prohibition on the tattoo of a person from another 'āiga including these designs. Tattoo subjects can also request specific designs, in order to show respect to particular matai to whose 'āiga the design is closely associated, to mark a special friendship with either their tattoo partner [soa] or some other friend, or for aesthetic or erotic reasons. One man, showing me his still healing tattoo, explained that a particular design on his thigh was a token of respect for the matai of a neighbouring village who had helped his 'āiga after the cyclone of 1989, one on his stomach was the design of the family of his closest male friend and the design around his penis was chosen to make his penis look like it was flying above his body. In contrast, siapo [bark cloth] designs are owned by 'āiga, and even by specific family lines within 'āiga and are associated with the female line of descent. No other 'āiga can legitimately use these designs on their bark cloth, a material which is used today only in formal exchanges between very high ranking matai.[3]

The tattoos are created by a specialist known as a *tufuga*, the same name applied to the circumcision specialist. Tattoos and circumcisions may be carried out by the same man, but this is not the rule. Quite often a *tufuga* will specialize in one process or the other. As well, *tufuga* may be noted for their particular skills in producing certain designs and chosen because of this. In pre-European Samoa, the *tufuga tatau* [tattoo specialist] may also have been an important advisor to the paramount *matai* of his family or district [Franco 1991:128-134]. Today there are very few *tufuga* in Samoa, although in recent years their number appears to have increased, as more and more younger Samoans seek "traditional" tattoos. Contemporary tattooists are respected for their skills, and no longer serve any other function with relation to *matai*.

The tattoos are created by hammering ink made from coconut charcoal into the skin with a set of up to six various sized mallets, made from bamboo sticks to which are attached combs of varying sizes, edged with pigs' teeth or bits of human bone. Today some *tufuga* use shards of glass, or small pieces of razor blades or other sharp metal in their combs, although combs made of pig teeth or human bone are highly prized. The mallets are not sacred objects, and should one break, it is simply discarded. The entire process, from outlining the designs, to the final filling in of the patterns, can take as long as a week, depending on the stamina of the subject, who determines how much of the design is completed at each session.

This is a painful process, in particular in the marking of designs over bones close to the surface of the skin. The persons being tattooed, most often *soa* partners, are also accompanied by other close friends who assist in the process, holding the arms and legs of the man being tattooed to prevent slipping, and telling stories or singing songs to amuse the men undergoing the process .

> *Tu'ufau, mai ali'i ē!*
> *'A'o le tu mai ea a le vavau.*
> *Te saga oi oe, 'a e pese a'u:*
> *E tupu le fafine fanau,*
> *E tupu le tane tā le tatau…*

> Relax, O Sir!
> This is an old time custom.
> You groan continually, but I sing:
> The woman must bear children,
> The man must be tattooed…

As well, villagers will often come and stand outside the house in which the tattoos are being done, voicing encouragement and approval as the de-

signs emerge, or as the young men successfully complete the more difficult and painful marking of complex designs.

Male tattooing appears, at least in some way, to be a parallel to either
childbirth or menstruation, and possibly both. The pain, the shedding of
blood—though not, I think, the blood itself—and the way the tattoo ra-
diates outward from the core of the body covering the generative parts of
the body in a cultured and unsheddable sheath, is striking for it similarity
to pregnancy as an embodied experience. Many of my informants said
things which might be summed up as "this is our answer to childbirth."
However, pressed on this, I found no consistency in the ideas connecting
tattooing with parturition. However, at the risk of mapping my own aesthetic judgement on these often allusive and vague comments, the connection is sufficiently reasonable to warrant further study. Like so much related to gender and sexing, this issue is more vexing, paradoxical and
puzzling than it first appears.

The self reported objective for receiving a tattoo is to demonstrate and
produce strong bodies. Enduring the tattoo process shows to the people
watching, and continues to show throughout the person's life, that he is
able to tolerate pain because a key aspect of Samoan strength is the ability to withstand long term physical discomfort. At the same time, the
process of tattooing creates strength in the individual being tattooed by
teaching his body its limits of endurance and tolerance. Finally, through
his body, the tattooed man constitutes the value and pursuit of strength
for the people around him.

This is one aspect of the embodiment of discipline. Another relates tattooing to the structures of authority within which Samoan bodies are deployed. A formal body tattoo is most often initiated by the subject's father,
always a *matai*. The father presents the idea of the tattoo to his son, who
has the right to refuse without explanation. If the son accepts, he is acknowledging a formal position of service to *matai* authority, through a public expression of service to his father's title and, through that, to all *matai*. After
acquiring a full tattoo, the son adopts certain patterns of submission and restraint. He becomes a kind of specialist servant to his father, the *matai*, carrying out his orders, acting on his behalf as a *'ava* preparer at important
fono, and comporting himself in sexual matters with dignity and constraint.
While not in fact a virgin, he is in significance one. His sexual or erotic body
becomes split from his adolescent, exploratory, body, strategically emerging,
when appropriate, as one or the other. At the same time the tattooed body
becomes a signifier of discipline itself, such as when a man raises his *lavalava*
to expose his tattoo as a signal to a group of boys misbehaving on a village
road of the authority that attaches to the *matai* and those who serve for him.

The tattooed man is a body enacting the disciplines of humility in the
presence of authority. There is dignity in his comportment while receiv-

ing the tattoo and, afterwards, a new modesty, because once tattooed, the body is figuratively, and literally, never again naked. This painful and selective act of embodiment, although changing in contemporary Samoa, still retains its disciplinary effect, and the willingness and ability of any person to undergo tattooing is afforded great honour and deference. As one elderly man told me, "to receive the tattoo, and to show it proudly, is to remind us all what is the truth of Samoa."

As I noted in Chapter 3, tattooing may have been related to chiefly status in a very direct way, in pre-European Samoa. All *matai* are said to have had full body tattoos, and indeed, early accounts suggest one could not be a *matai* without a tattoo. The principles of service and humility which the tattoo enacts were the same, but they were more directly linked to the ultimate acquisition of chiefly status in Samoa. Like all historical reconstructions, however, this is tentative and speculative. Today, many Samoans find the use of a tattoo as a device for claiming authority, troubling, and inappropriate. "A man who has a tattoo so he can be a prince," one man told me, "is covering his body with a very bad tattoo. Tattoos make you strong, and make you humble, and they remind us that to be a good Samoan is to be strong and humble and to serve your *'āiga* and your *matai*." Unlike mass, which I suggested in Chapter 3 some *matai* may be appropriating as a way of marking their distinctiveness as members of a fixed class, tattooing has been appropriated by younger, and mostly untitled, Samoans, explicitly as a means, for many, of indicating their commitment to traditions of service and propriety.

Where tattooing is a special form of disciplined body through which docility and strength are enacted, circumcision [*tafao*] is a generic form of body discipline which every boy is obligated to undertake. Girls, however, do not undergo any form of organized scarring or body modification as they grow up. As one woman put it to me, "is *mai masina* [menstruation] not enough for that."

Circumcision is initiated voluntarily by boys anywhere from the age of 6 onward. With his *soa* partner, the boys will approach their mothers to ask them to make arrangements for the *tufuga* to visit the village to perform the ceremony. This inverts the role the father may play in tattooing, where he approaches his son, but in each case the decision is the boys, and not the parents. While many years separate the two events, in both cases it is the boy himself who judges if he is ready and able to sustain the operations. One of the mothers would then contact a specialist in circumcision. Gifts of food and fine mats are given to the specialist, although this is not a payment, and may be refused. Rather, it is a gift for a gift, fine mats given in exchange for the *tufuga* giving back to the mother a strong son. Today, while a small percentage of circumcisions are performed by *tufuga*, most are performed by a travelling clinic staffed by a Western trained doctor, which visits each village at least once a year. Young boys who have requested *tafao* are then circumcised together in a group.

On the day of the circumcision, the boys say goodbye to their fathers in the early morning hours and spend the remainder of the day with their mothers. Today this can be quite a large group of mothers and their sons. The boys are bathed thoroughly in fresh water, and provided with new *lavalava*, which they do not yet put on. They are taken by their mothers to the *fale* where the operation will take place, naked and laughing boisterously. Usually the highest ranking boy will go first. From the moment he enters the house, the other boys become quiet, only occasionally talking among themselves. The procedure today involves the complete excision of the prepuce, without the aid of anaesthetics and usually without post operative suturing. It takes a few brief moments. The physician, who now replaces the *tufuga* in almost all cases, makes two simple incisions in the foreskin, cutting between them with surgical scissors. Some young men still have this form of *tafao*, and one adolescent boy from a village where I worked showed me his "real Samoan *tafao*" with great pride.

During the procedure, and following it, the boy is silent. After the excision is complete, he walks with his mother from the *fale*, and sits with her to one side of the group of waiting boys. After the final boy is finished, the entire group travels, either on foot or by truck if necessary, to the sea. Here the boys bathe repeatedly in the salt water. While their first venture into the ocean is somewhat quiet and apprehensive, the bathing soon turns into a boisterous game, the boys racing each other in and out of the water. At the end of this bathing, which can last all afternoon, the boys are handed their new *lavalava*, which they now put on, tying them in the front knotted manner in which men are expected to tie this garment, in contrast to the side knotting manner in which women wear theirs. From this point on they are required to always wear their *lavalava* in this way. While visiting an outer village I witnessed an older *matai* stopping several young boys with their *lavalava* knotted to the side and, with a stick, lifting their dress to see if any had already been circumcised. Only one boy had, the others still too young, and his family was fined a small amount of food for the boy's transgression.

On the boys' return to the village, people will call congratulations as the boys walk by. The boys are treated to special food, including portions or dishes usually reserved for *matai* or for high ranking guests, before retiring early to rest. No other special treatment, other than repeated individual ocean baths, is given to the healing of the remains of the foreskin. Infection is surprisingly rare given the tendency of sores to suppurate in the tropics.

When asked why they had decided to ask for *tafao*, most boys told me that they felt it was now time to begin to become strong. The act of circumcision, in which no effort is made to ensure comfort or to minimize pain, is a marker of an emerging transition in a boy's body, from the condition of relative weakness and softness in childhood, to the strength and endurance associated with adult bodies. It is also a trigger which begins a new phase in the boy's growth, marked by increasing concern with his ability to demonstrate his strength. Following circumcision, he does not take on new duties, but now, when he carries out his work around the household, he is expected to do so with the same stamina and vigour as boys twice his age. So strong is this association between *tafao* and strength as a virtue of full personhood, that the single most offensive insult you can pay to a man is the epithet "*kefe,*" the informal pronunciation of the vulgar word *tefe* [circumcision], which translates as "get circumcised."

Circumcision, like tattooing, locates the body in a field of discipline and service. By altering the body, in both private and public manners, the boys are engaging in the process of creating with their flesh the principles of endurance, responsibility, obedience, and propriety, which are the hallmarks of the disciplined Samoan body. Like the array of bodies in the *fono*, and the service of the *tāupou* in the *'ava* ceremony, the bodies of recently circumcised boys engage in a lived experiential way the constitution of these principles. Bodies are enactments of culture in their movement and postures, their alterations and sensations. The boys bathing in the sea are feeling and doing discipline and order in the sting of the salt water in their proudly acquired wounds.

Correcting Bodies: Possession and Punishment

Wounding the body is also central to formal acts of punishment and discipline in Samoa. The abjection of the body, the denial of its humanness, and the infliction of often severe injury, are characteristic of formal forms of punishment and discipline. I mentioned the potential brutality of physical punishment of older children at the beginning of this chapter. I want to consider some more formal aspects of punishment and discipline now.

There are several different sources of punishment in Samoa, including *matai* or the *fono* as a whole, parents, church leaders, the police and courts, and *aitu*, the malicious spirits who are everywhere in Samoa. I will only consider the embodying implications of two here, *matai* and *aitu* because these are the most common forms of discipline and punishment in everyday life.

Aitu are either spirit beings in their own right, or the spirits of dead ancestors, or the hand servants of the spirits of dead ancestors.[4] The most dangerous class of *aitu* are known as *teine*. *Teine* are vicious female *aitu* who are associated, most often, with bodies of water on the islands. They are notorious for seducing young men in their sleep (the evidence of which is the evidence of nocturnal emissions) and for possessing young girls. Saumaiafe is a particularly mean *aitu*. I witnessed her interference with two girls in my home village in Samoa. The girls in question first became listless and disobedient, and refused to rise from their sleeping mats in the morning to perform their chores, or care for their younger siblings. A few days after this began, they were seen walking through the village with red earth smeared in their hair. Red is the colour of Saumaiafe, who delights in sitting in the highest limbs of trees, holding her head off her shoulders, and combing her long red hair. This red earth in the girl's hair signalled to everyone in the village that Saumaiafe was at work and steps were immediately taken to deal with her presence. This involved bringing in a possession specialist, a *taulāaitu* or medium, adept at speaking with Saumaiafe, in order to determine the cause of this possession. The girls were examined and their families interviewed. In each case a social cause, the malfeasance of another family member who had offended the *aitu*, was determined to be the reason for the possession, and, after the offenders made public apologies, both girls recovered.

In another case of possession, one in which I was actually called upon to help rid the girl of the tormenting *teine*, it transpired that the girl was being punished for having sex with a boy who was too closely related to her. Finally, Saumaiafe was implicated in the death of two young women, and the disfiguring injury of a young man, when she caused a small four wheel drive vehicle to overturn on a winding cross island road. In the weeks that followed the accident, it emerged that the girls had been involved in a scheme to steal from a church after the regular Sunday collection. Because the church was in a village adjacent to the sliding rock pool where Saumaiafe lived, she had become incensed at the young people, and had killed them.

Aitu punishment is usually not as dramatic as these incidents. More often it involves being tripped or hit and occasionally entered by the *aitu*, each of which can cause injury or illness. It is also not necessarily enacted on the specific offender in a family. As often as not, *aitu* will attack some other, usually weaker, family member, including unborn children. Significant birth defects, such as Down's Syndrome, dwarfism, or improperly formed limbs, are often attributed to *aitu* attacks as a form of punishment of one or both of the parents, or of some relative close to them, who has offended an *aitu*. This choice of victim in *aitu* punishment reinforces the mutuality of blame and responsibility in wrongdoing across a wide network of particular people. *Aitu* occupy and police the dangerous space of the bush, and the secret places in the village where offense and crimes may take place. They are an important source of discipline and punishment, attacking the body as an exercise in social control.

The human-directed forms of punishment are also primarily focused on the abjection of the body. Banishment is the most serious form of punishment, short of capital punishment, which is rare. A man, and his immediate household, are stripped of almost all of their possessions, and forced to leave the village. Because of patterns of obligation between nearby villages, the family are forced to wander, *ta'a*, the animal condition of aimless roaming. In some instances of banishment, the family has perished because they were unable to find a new village to live in not obligated to the authority of the banishing village. Today banishment is illegal in Samoa, but it is still practiced, occasionally resulting in the members of the banishing *fono* being charged in criminal court, and punished as well. I am familiar with three cases of banishment in which the court punished the *matai* who issued the order of banishment. In each case, the family did not return to the village from which they had been shunned. When I spoke with members of two of the banished families, I was told that they felt the decision was fair and just, and that they would abide by the order, no matter what the police did to the *matai*. Indeed, one man from a banished family went so far as to appear at the trial of one of the *matai* who had banished him to plead with the court to not interfere with the *matai's* decision.

Other forms of physical punishment also denature the body and render it less than human. A man can be trussed like a pig and burned in an open *umu*, in the manner in which pigs are cooked prior to ceremonial exchange. Being tied in the area beneath a house where pigs sleep, or being tossed food scraps like a dog, are other formal forms of physical punishment, combined with beatings, having small bones broken, being stripped naked and forced to walk through the village, and being made to smear your body with pig or dog faeces and then lay prostrate on the ground begging forgiveness. Early in 1994 a *matai* was killed by members of his *'āiga*. All the members of his extended family entered his house and several shot him. This happened because of his failure to fulfil his duties as the family's head, his mistreatment of family members, who he had used as free labour in his business, and his misappropriation of ceremonial exchange goods for his own use. While there is a general code of crime and appropriate punishment, the application of a given punishment is determined, not by the abstract nature of the crime itself, but by the constellation of events, relationships, and obligations in which the offender and the offended are located. It is not likely that a person would be executed for stealing a pig, but it is also not impossible for this to occur.

Punishment can be avoided, or suspended, if the offender takes the initiative and abjects themself in a ritual known as *ifoga*. The head of a family charged with some serious offence, such as the theft of pigs or murder [Shore 1982:19], presents himself on the *malae* of the village of the offended person, and lays prostrate on the ground before the *fale* of the offended *matai*, draping himself in fine mats of special quality and value. At regular intervals he calls out from beneath his sheath of mats to be allowed to come forward and plead forgiveness. This can go on for several days before his presence is acknowledged by the *matai* of the offended family. In some cases, the *matai* performing *ifoga* will remain through the night, but most often he withdraws, never showing himself from under his pile of mats, to return in the morning and repeat the process.

In *ifoga*, the body of a high ranking person is completely subsumed by the web of obligation and allegiance embodied in the fine mats beneath which he cowers. All the attachments of authority and power which his body instantiates in other circumstances evaporate in the air that carries his abjected plea for forgiveness and reintegration. *Ifoga* is the site of the greatest danger in restoring social order in Samoa, because in the degradation of the *matai* beneath his mats the entire structure of Samoan authority, as it is enacted in the presence of the body of the *matai*, is imperiled. Ultimately, *ifoga* works because, as several *matai* explained after having accepted the apology of a man whose three sons had gangraped a young boy, to refuse the apology of a *matai* "would destroy him and maybe then it would destroy us. It would be showing off to refuse to say that you [the offender] must now come back inside the house." At risk in *ifoga* are the entire panoply of associations between dignity, authority, co-operation, and the body, which are the key components of Samoan humanness.

In this sense then, *ifoga* inverts the other instantiation of the powerful body of the *matai*, which takes place during the *saofa'i*, or investiture of a *matai*. After deliberation by the extended family, agreement is reached about the conferring of a title on to a specific man or woman. The ritual through which this conferral occurs involves the stripping and redressing of the newly titled person in traditional cloths and clothing as a way of signifying his or her transformation from solely a participant in *Fa'a Samoa* to a special kind of body which also carries it. The body of the *matai* is masked with bark cloth and fine mats, a covering which renounces the *matai*'s own body in favour of a new body which is never quite singular again. And like the covering of the body of the *matai* during the *ifoga*, this covering of the newly titled man or woman locates the entire enactment of the values and prescriptions of *Fa'a Samoa* on the skin and in the bones of the *matai* as someone who now bears these values and prescriptions as a new kind skin. At stake in the *saofa'i* as in the *ifoga* are the core values of effacement and consensus through which individual bodies can be made to disappear, and because of which individual bodies become the entire culture and community of which they are, in other circumstances, only a functional part.

Disciplining and de-humanizing the body are inseparable qualities of Samoan social control. The prison explicitly treats the inmates as animals, providing them with none of the comforts of humanness, from the abysmal quality of the food to the filth and lack of excretory privacy of the cell areas. Insults, such as telling someone they "fuck like a dog," or the epithet *kefe* [get circumcised], with its implications that the body of the insulted person is a weak, animal body, and not worth human consideration, also contribute to the everyday abjection of the social body in discipline and punishment.

What this produces is a body protective of its humanity. It is a body which strives to enact the signal qualities of dignity, humility, and strength, which are central to embodiment in Samoa. This is not a docile and submissive body, but an active one, actively pursuing recognition as truly human and as fully Samoan. Abjection is something one guards against and something, when it happens, one accepts, and acts to overcome. The body punished is the body denied good and proper social meaning. It is a body mortified and then revitalized in apology and forgiveness.

Foucault's docile bodies on the assembly line, or in the prison wards, are not the same bodies one finds in the surveilled and abjecting arena of formal social control in Samoa. The Foucauldian objective of discipline, a body seen in all its aspects, and restrained and denied, is not the Samoan objective of discipline. Where power travels downward from the panoptic gaze of Foucault's mechanisms of power, in Samoa power travels through the field of embodiment like an energizing current, sustaining the body as a site and cause of propriety. In enacting discipline and punishment, as in pursuing sexual partners, or feasting to excess, or playing rugby into the early hours of night, Samoans do not submit to power, they participate in it, in the manner and form in which their bodies are invented and deployed in the field of responsibility and obligation, a system tense with anxiety, ambiguity, and risk. The limits and the expanses of pleasure—the rugby games and the rites of courtship—are what I turn to now.

Chapter 7

Pleasures and Punishments: Living in and Beyond the Appropriate

Virtue is something lofty, elevated and regal...Pleasure is something lowly and servile...Virtue you will meet in the temple, the forum and the senate house...Pleasure you will find lurking and hanging around in the shadows, round the baths and saunas...

Seneca

Foucault, in *Discipline and Punish*, writes of the "policy of coercion that acts upon the body, a calculated manipulation of its elements, its gestures, its behaviours...a machinery of power that explores it, breaks it down and rearranges it" [1979:137]. The body, for Foucault, is a "political anatomy" and a "mechanics of power" [p.138]. The objective of this micro-physics of body constraint is docility, a body rendered visible in a field of power and social imprisonment. The body is abjected by the orders of power that surround it.

This point towards a dynamic tension which exists between the embodiment of experience, and the orders of social stability and meaning within which this experience is carried out. In this chapter I explore some of the sites and practices in which Samoan bodies are deployed in pleasure and discipline, compliance and disobedience, and about how the body is implicated in the process of creating an orderly and meaningful everyday life.

This is especially important in a society where ranking and status are as formalized as they are in Samoa, every member of a community stands in relationships of discipline to almost every other member of the community, extending not only through the person's *'āiga*, but throughout the entire country. This question of who must obey who, under what circumstances, and to what extent, is a constant in everyone's life. Illustrated in Figure 7.1, this is a complicated and complicating system of often competing individuals and institutions with different interests, and often conflicting interests.[1] Cross cutting this are obligations of kinship, familial obligations

131

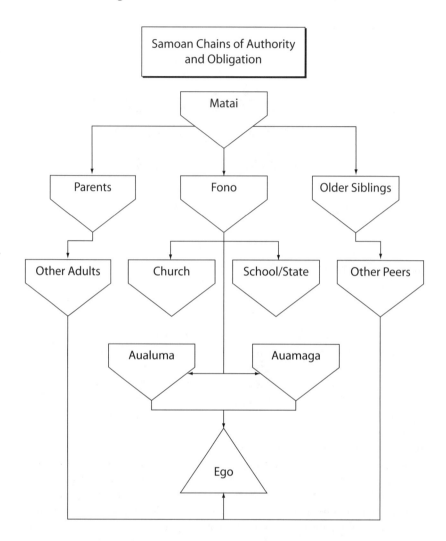

Figure 7.1 Samoans maneuver within a web of authority
and submission with multiple and multiplying levels.

to siblings and parents, obligations to *matai*, all of which shift and change, and as often as not become positions of authority rather than submission. A command from one authority can be superseded by a command from another, and obligations to one powerful figure can be overruled by obligations to some other. As such, obedience in any context is premised on a calculation of how accepting the authority of person X relates to, and effects, conditions of obligation and obedience to persons Y and Z. At the same time, this web of potential sites of command and obedience opens up a wide field of strategic disobedience, so obeying is never simply submission, but needs to be seen more conditionally as an agreement to submit, for now. Discipline plays out in and amongst these multiplying structures. Later in this chapter I will explore how this effects the enactment of sexual behaviour as an embodying praxis. For now, I want to draw the readers attention to the web of interests and structures in which the embodiment of propriety and obedience are carried out. Obedience in Samoa can see best described as a conversation, an open ended mechanics of negotiation, rather than a simple submission to authority and domination. Because of the rich structure of allegiance and compliance in which each Samoan finds him or herself discipline and obedience are something done with and through the body, and not something simply done to the body [cf Foucault 1979].

Even imprisonment by the courts, as Shore [1977, 1982] notes, is practiced as a negotiation between who has the authority to command and how those commands relate to the webs of obligation, and negotiated compliance, in which the commanded person lives. Both the commanding person and the person being commanded participate in these negotiations. Each side understands that the successful and legitimate sentence reinstates a proper understanding of, and balance between, an individual's multiple connections of obedience. "It is good that I go to prison," one man told me, "because [my punishment] makes my family a full family again, makes it alright for me to go home into my family again." Samoans rarely give in, they give over, selectively and strategically.

The conversational quality of obedience can be see in even everyday events, exemplified in the processes of saying, hearing, and failing to here orders and commands. Obedience is *fa'alogo*, which means, literally, to hear or pay attention to. To obey is to hear and understand what is being said. As such, very young children are not expected to obey, because they have yet to learn the meaning of words and speech acts. Once a child can speak and understand, it is obligated to obey. However, rules of speaking, and in particular rules ensuring that you are understood, leave a space around commands where misunderstanding can be manipulated as a strategy of refusal. In Samoa, persons of higher status are, by virtue of their status, not expected to initiate what linguists call clarification sequences [Ochs 1988:128-144], speech acts in which speakers engage in strategies through which an initial utterance is restated, explained, or enhanced, to clarify its meaning. At the same time, persons of status lower than the speaker are culturally prohibited from requiring clarification by the higher status person. Inversely, it is inappropriate for a person of higher status to require a person of lower status to repeat what they have said since, to admit failure to hear would be an admission of immodesty, that is, a failure to pay appropriate attention. When Samoans engage in clarification sequences they adopt what Ochs calls the minimal grasp strategy, deliberately "pretending" to not have heard anything the speaker has said in the hopes the speaker will repeat him or herself [1988:132]. They avoid the other common clarification sequence, the expressed guess strategy, in which the hearer repeats to the speaker what he thinks the speaker has said as a way of triggering clarification since, as Ochs notes, to do so would be to presume in a public way to be able to see what the other person is thinking or feeling, something Samoans avoid doing [see also Gerber 1975; Clement 1974]. The affect of this dispreference for seeking clarification is a space of misunderstanding which can be used as a strategy in itself. Within the multiple and depending on the circumstances, multiplying network of interests, authorities and obligations, the tactic of deliberately not hearing is a powerful one giving auditors some control over how they are controlled, and restraining the untrammelled imposition of authority and command by institutionalizing a mechanism which necessarily transforms orders into something closer to requests.

Within these conditioning practices and strategies, Samoans engage in processes of discipline and pleasure, compliance and collaboration. The body is the central locus of these processes.

Cooperation and Surveillance

Early in my stay in Samoa, I sat one morning on the stoop of my house, after a night of nausea and pain. Louisa, who, I learned later, was my aunt, came by my house with a small bundle of flowers. Before she could say anything I vomited noisily. As she reached over to wipe my face with the hem of her *lavalava,* she said, "*mālō le pua'iga,*" which, I found out from someone later, meant literally "well done the vomiting." This is an example of a *mālō* exchange, which have the form of "well done" [the action] said by an observer, answered with *mālō le tapua'i* [well done the support] by the actor. This form of encouragement, of a kind of shared responsibility or cooperation in everyday life, is a key aspect of Samoan interaction [Ochs1988:207-8]. Cooperation is important in all activities. It is a cooperation which makes the spectator a participant. Encouraging a young man chopping to pieces the huge breadfruit tree, which had collapsed across the road in front of my house during a cyclone, is as important a form of support and joint effort as taking up an axe, and joining him in the actual hacking.

Samoan action is a complicated tangle of collaboration, sympathy, mutual assistance and encouragement, and obedience and deference. In a sense, Samoans never do anything on their own. This is exemplified in *mālō* exchanges. Driving a friend between Apia and the airport, I drove carefully around some badly damaged tar seal, avoiding the worst of the potholes. My friend turned to me and said, *"mālō le fa'auli"* [well done the driving.]. My Samoan father returned from attending a funeral in American Samoa. As he got out of the taxi, his oldest son called to him *"mālō malaga"* [well done the journey] to which Sei'a replied, *"mālō le fa'amuli"* [well done the staying behind]. In these exchanges, which form an idiom of everyday talk, Samoans enact their experience and understanding that all actions are connected in a mutual relationship of support and responsibility.

The *mālō* exchanges embody a connection between humility and co-operation, with no actor taking all the credit, and no spectator ever completely absolved or removed from the actions he or she witnesses. "Well done the tree climbing" enacts recognition of a job well done, while "well done the support" recognizes that no action is possible without *tapua'i*, that is, without support. Obedience and deference, taken together with this sense of interpenetrating cooperation, concatenate and combine all bodies, and all actions, in a single network of common purpose and responsibility. Whenever you meet someone along the road, the convention is to say hello, the form of which is simply *malo*. The link between this form of *malo* and the supportive form well done [*mālō*] was understood by my informants as a form of contraction of the long vowel form. *Malo* is an abbreviated form of *mālō*, a constant and inescapable reminder of the links between all members of the community.

It is impossible, therefore, to grasp obedience in Samoa without recognizing this intersubjective web from which no act can be extricated. In the connection between watching and joint responsibility, the spaces of good and bad behaviour connect in the constant vigilance and cooperation of day to day life.

In my discussion of village layout in Chapter 3, I made the point that village design involves a "sacred" open space [*malae*] surrounded by the household lots of village members. All important social activity takes place on the *malae*, in full view of all village households. In the wall-less traditional households, all the activities of daily family life are visible to the entire village. In circles of decreasing dignity extending around the *malae* and household ring, surveillance and sociality also decrease until, at the civilized fringes of the bush, the locus occupied by *aitu* and dangerous animals, social visibility is conceptually, and practically, nil.[2]

However, in speaking of the visible and invisible in Samoa it is helpful to distinguish different kinds of privacy, because in each case a different kind of invisibility is being enacted. Deception [*fa'ase'e*] refers to things done to trick and harm someone. This includes actions done away from view such as stealing. It also includes actions committed which impersonate good action in order to mask a harmful one, such as claiming to be a relative when one is not, or impersonating a *matai*. In contrast, secrecy [*mealilo*], refers to things which, legitimately, others should not see or hear, such as ritual secrets surrounding the investiture of *matai*. Finally, the word for privacy [*totinō*] connects the word body [*tinō*] with such concepts as kinship, intimacy and propriety. It refers to such things as sex, intimate conversation, and other close, personal interactions.[3]

These three types of invisibility apply to different areas of social life. However, they have undergone a significant transformation in Samoan's perceptions of changes in their society. In traditional villages, surveillance was extensive. That is, it took in the entire range of seeable activities as a web of related actions. Every individual action could be seen in relation to all other actions in the village, and the individual actor was not so much the focus of surveillance as he or she was a component of a wide ranging and all encompassing gaze [Keene 1978]. Changes in village layout, and in particular the development of isolated household compounds, and the fragmentation of the *malae*, have made surveillance in village life more ambiguous. While villages have retained their conceptual geography of dignified and undignified space, physical changes have also located asocial or dangerous acts in the village core. The peripheral, dark spaces have been compressed inward into the village centre by population pressures, which have swallowed up plantation land between villages. Ruth, an older woman, once told me that when she was a girl "lovers doing sex was funny because we would see it in the bush sometimes after evening church and we would throw stones at them and laugh, and no one would get angry, but today people want to stop all the things boys and girls [teenagers] do because now it is here beside us, beside where we eat and pray." The periphery and the core are now less readily distinguished. As a result, there has been an increase in what I call intensive surveillance, which, echoing Foucault, applies to all acts

> a micro-penalty of time [lateness, absences, interruptions of tasks], of activity [inattention, lack of zeal], of behaviour [impoliteness, disobedience] of speech [idle chatter, indolence] of the body [incorrect attitudes, irregular gestures, lack of cleanliness], of sexuality [impurity, indecency]...making the slightest departures from correct behaviour subject to punishment. [Foucault 1979:178, cited in Synnott 1993:229, brackets in original].

Older Samoans often mention increases in gossip, increased interference by family members, and an increased awareness of being scrutinized. One man, frustrated because our conversation was continually interrupted by people wanting to know who I was, told me that there is no time for intimacy [*fa'auō*, referring to actions between close friends] today because everyone is looking in your doors to see what you are doing. Before you would walk through a village and know what was happening without looking, without even seeing, but now it is too noisy and there is too much looking and asking. The village has become a place for gossip and spying...everyone is always staring inside at everyone else.

Many Samoans feel there has been a significant decrease in privacy in what, on the surface at least, appears to have been the most open and immodest social geography imaginable, a circular village of houses without walls. Walls have created smaller and smaller intimate spaces, because they have increased the range of private spaces and brought activities, once reserved for the dark, periphery right outside the front door. Today village paths and roadways can be defined as *aga*, socially good, and *lēaga*, bad or dangerous, depending on what is being done on them, and by whom, complicating and rendering the meaning of public and private space flexible, and at the same time, stressful and tense by intensifying the controlling function of the social gaze at the heart of village life. The modern Samoan village remains a carefully modulated geography of visibility and invisibility but changes in village layout, while retaining the traditional conceptual frame, have altered the way that frame of surveillance is experienced, and have rendered it more vexatious and even more dangerous. Many people told me that the modern village with its competing and ill defined pathways had led to increased movement of *aitu* within the villages themselves, and it is apparent from comments like "I know longer know where it is good to shit," that this increasingly stressful moral geography is directly affecting the way people navigate around the demands of embodied presence and propriety. As such, bodies deployed in the village space are constantly shifting and changing as the nature of the space they are moving in shifts and changes. On this ground, framed by formality, cooperation and obedience, and the ambiguity of private space, Samoans deploy their formal bodies in play and work.

* * *

Fights, Games, and Work: Aspects of Co-operation and Support

A fight broke out at the Lalaga Night Club in Fugalei, one of the 11 contiguous villages which make up the formal Apia town area. Boys from the village of Vaimoso chased a group of boys from the village of Matautu out into the bar's small parking lot where a melee ensued that left three people with broken bones, a car on fire, and several windows in the bar owner's house broken. I was woken in the middle of the night by the sound of the Vaimoso boys returning along the main village road, talking and laughing, walking behind a pickup truck in which one of them lay unconscious, and bleeding from a gash on his thigh. A soft voice whispered my name from outside my window. I lit the hurricane lamp beside my sleeping mat to see several faces peering in at me.

"Douglass, can you bring some medicine to tie up Tone's leg, he has a cut," a voice asked through the window of my bedroom.

"A bad cut?" I asked, thinking quickly about my St. John's Ambulance training 20 years earlier.

"No, Douglass, a good cut, a good strong cut."

The rest of the night was spent applying compresses to Tone's leg and listening to the now sobering boys tell, over and over, the story of the fight with the Matautu boys, and the preservation of the honour of Vaimoso. It turned out Tone had been drinking heavily through most of the evening and was extremely drunk by the later hours of the night. He had stumbled against a table at which a group of Matautu residents, both male and female, had been sitting and in the act, had knocked a large pitcher of water over on to one of the women's laps. The men at the table had risen to confront Tone, but the press on the dance floor directly beside them had swallowed him up. Sometime later, a smaller group of Matautu boys saw Tone sitting slumped in a chair at a deserted table. They surrounded him, and kicked him to the ground, shouting that Vaimoso boys were animals who did not know how to behave in front of their sisters. The Vaimoso boys who had been with Tone, saw this from across the bar and moved, as a group, to surround and then chase the other boys out of the bar. The fight ensued.

"You never kick someone who is drunk, do you?" one of the boys asked me.

"And Matautu is a pig path, not a real village. They said we did not know how to be with our sisters, when they fuck their sisters every morning before they fuck their pigs," another added.

"AFTER they fuck their pigs," another retorted.

The vitriol the Vaimoso boys expressed during that night was the most intensive example of expletive language I witnessed during my time in Samoa. While I found the sexual content of the images the boys used interesting, what was most striking to me about this fight, and the days that followed, is that the fighting and the injury were understood as fun and a part of being friends with the boys from the other village. It was part of a friendly competitiveness between the boys of Vaimoso, and the boys of

Matautu, in the cross island rugby tournament which was being played over the weeks in which this fight occurred.

Rugby is the national sport of Samoan men, taking over most villages in the hours just before the sun goes down. It is the one group activity which takes place on the *malae* without the direction and supervision of adults, and is considered by many to be an important training ground for the development of strong and capable bodies. It is a rough, and often very aggressive game and injuries are common, though rarely very serious. In this game specific objectives of both endurance and cooperation are embodied. The ability to play long and to run almost constantly over the course of a game, which may take several hours to play, is the mark of both a good rugby player, and a good healthy Samoan body. A good rugby player needs to be able to move the ball, to run longer and faster than members of the other team, and to know the fundamental value of teamwork. In playing well, the Samoan boy is not trying to excel personally, but to enhance the overall excellence of his team. One effect of this is that players with particular skills at scoring or passing do not try to perfect those skills, and are not assigned roles in the games related to their special skills. The game is shared. It is not unusual to see a team's finest ball handler pass the ball to another player, even when he has a clear and easy shot on the goal himself, because, as one boy explained, "Asovali has not had a try in too many games." That Asovali misses the goal, or is perhaps not even in a good position to score, is less important than the fact that, as a team member, he needs to be given his due opportunity to contribute.

Inter-team competition is framed by this internal cooperation, and so, inter-team competition is not simply about winning over some other group of boys. In the cross island rugby competition the co-operative qualities of the teams are pitted against each other. This intersection between the competition between teams and the co-operative character of team work conjoins in fights such as the one I described above. Fighting is a levelling strategy which constitutes cooperation and competition on the bodies in the fighting groups, in the same way that it is constituted in the rugby match. What is being enacted in the fight is a form of co-operative understanding about the nature of the teams as single connected units. In fighting, the boys are negotiating and enacting, with bruises and broken bones, a relationship of collusion between the two groups which constitutes the competitive relationship of the tournament as part of the more central co-operative processes which govern the teams arrayed against each other. The Vaimoso boys were both deploying and defending the honour of Vaimoso as a "true community," by directly confronting the Matautu boys, as a group, and reinforcing the importance of their own co-operative support. This fight, although disturbing to the owner of the bar, was not about antagonism and hatred, but was an enactment of the collaborative nature of embodiment as it is enacted in play. Like the rugby game itself, the fight was not about bodies butting up against each other as separate entities. It was about bodies colluding as parts of a unit which, in their engagement in the fight, re-asserted and enacted anew, that unitary cooperation.

In contrast, fights between individuals are defined as fundamentally *lēaga* and are heavily sanctioned, in the same way that showing off in a rugby game or other endeavour is sanctioned by insult or shunning. The strong body arrayed against some person or thing as a singular act of violence is an inappropriately strong body, and the teamwork of rugby, like the teamwork of legitimate group fighting, sites this distinction as central to the emerging development of the boys good and proper sense of their bodily presence in the community.

Fighting as part of a group, and team play, each enact two concerns: one for demonstrating strength, and the other for enacting and reinforcing the quality of each boy's commitment to group membership and group identity. As the Samoan proverb says, "first friends, then broken heads." Team play, and fighting between groups, engages the boy's bodies in the combined pursuit of humility and strength. These precepts legitimate the deployment of fighting or competing bodies in what are closely circumscribed spaces for such activities, because who and where play occurs is part of this process of appropriating space and enacting the cooperative obligations of *Fa'a Samoa*.

Earlier, I described the rings of decreasing dignity which form the conceptual geography of the village. The central space, the *malae* or its fragmented equivalent of internal village roads and paths, is the most dignified space of the village, and as such, it is also the most social and safe. The *malae* is the site of play, and other activities, which are social in their orientation. Figure 7.2 illustrates the relationship between body deployments in play, and other activities, and the dignity of socially ordered space.

The outer ring, the space of invisibility, is the space of solo play, away from the eyes of the village. Games like "truck," in which young children build ramshackle contraptions of sticks with *pisupo* tins for wheels, are something commonly played in the roadways around the plantations. Children will quietly push their trucks up and down the roadways, singing to themselves or telling themselves jokes. They even spend long afternoons on the plantation roads with their trucks talking to themselves about events in the village, about episodes in their households, or about their day at school. Another favourite activity while playing with their trucks is to practice their English, away from the correcting presence of adults. Older boys will practice with their rugby balls by themselves, and older girls will often spend time in this "solo" space weaving plaits of palm leaves into vague doll figures, an activity I never once saw anyone do in the village proper. In the household circle, the ring within the periphery in which, ei-

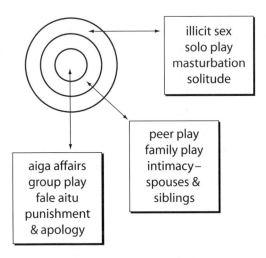

illicit sex
solo play
masturbation
solitude

peer play
family play
intimacy –
spouses &
siblings

aiga affairs
group play
fale aitu
punishment
& apology

Figure 7.2 Space, Dignity and Activity in Samoan Villages

ther physically or conceptually, the households are arrayed around the *malae*, play in the form of either dyadic peer play, or play among siblings, is most common. Children will play together with their trucks, or chase each other around their houses, laughing and shouting. Older young persons will gather in small groups of three or four peers to sing or play guitar. Adult men will spend their evenings playing the national card game, *suipi*. Women get together in small groups in each others' *fale*, to weave sleeping mats, or to talk. On the *malae* proper, games are group events, team oriented and co-operative activities complete with supporting spectators and, as I described above for the rugby teams, unified corporate teams enacting and reinforcing their relationships of support.

The closer to the *malae* one comes in observing village play, the greater the sociability and dignity of the playing bodies present. The bodies deployed in the periphery are individual, disconnected bodies. As one moves deeper into the core of the village, the individual body begins to disappear, replaced by bodies arrayed in relationships of either communal pursuit or cooperative effort. Finally, on the *malae*, the bodies deployed are invisible as singular entities, replaced by their part in the cooperative whole. There is an intensification of connection, from the random and individualized disconnections of bodies in the periphery, through the intimate connections of spouses, parents and children, and siblings and peers, in the household circle, to the self-effacing web of connection among all members of the community enacted on the *malae*.

A similar pattern is apparent in the kinds of work which are carried out in the various rings of dignity in the village. Plantation work, carried out on the outskirts of the villages, and often quite some distance from them, is highly individualized, depending on the individuals qualities of strength and endurance. As we move into the household circle, we still find activities performed based on specific qualities, but now in terms of generic qualities such as gender. Women weave mats and men boil the white food. Women clean the house, while men clean the *paepae*, the roughly paved area around the family house. Added to this, however, is a cooperative or joint component as well. Groups of cooperating individuals carry out the work in the household circle, the single working body of the boy in the plantation replaced by linked bodies functioning as a unit in the pursuit of tasks. At the border between the household ring ['*aufale*] and the *malae*, the work of greatest dignity is carried out. For women, this work is the weaving of *ie toga*, the fine mats exchanged between 'āiga at special events, such as weddings and funerals. This work is reserved for the oldest and highest status women, and is a major point of connection between the deployment of their labouring bodies, and the system of rank, authority, and cooperation within which village life occurs. For men, and in particular for men of rank, the most dignified labour in the village is actually as a kind of janitor, both *tulafale* and *ali'i* taking great pride in sweeping the roadways of the villages, often with the help of younger boys, and in the case of the villages where I spent the most time, almost always accompanied by a pail of weak '*ava*, a mild intoxicant about which I will say more shortly. The most dignified labour of all is in the form of the *fono*, the meetings of *matai* to discuss village and family affairs, which usually take place in the meeting house of the paramount 'āiga of the village. This is the work of both men and women, and as we shall see shortly, also the most dignified work of the young and untitled. The fono is the most observed and open of formal communal activities, with non-*matai* villagers often surrounding the meeting house to watch, and listen to the proceedings.

The connection of bodies in conjoint efforts is not the only aspect of embodiment implicated in this pattern of activities. Movement, a key aspect of deployment, is also involved. Proper movement in Samoa is slow, steady, and stately. Rushing, extreme exertion, and frenetic activity, are avoided, because they are seen as showing off. The deeper one moves into the village proper, the more restrained movement becomes until, at the point of connection between '*aufale* and *malae*, movement comes to a complete stop, exemplified in the rigid posture of *matai* in meetings, or women sitting crosslegged weaving mats.

This combination of the embodied Samoan as someone who works according to roles and obligations, and the embodied Samoan as someone who plays within these same rules, comes together most explicitly in the *fale'aitu*, comedy performances put on by village groups on the *malae* on weekend evenings. The *fale'aitu* is a carnivalesque space of inversion, where authority is made the subject of jokes, and where the lowest in status are accorded the power to criticize, and make light of, the fundamental ordering principles of *fa'a Samoa* [Bahktin 1984]. *Fale'aitu* take the form of skits performed, in costumes, by villagers. The content of the skits is often ribald, and is always insulting toward the figures of authority in the village or district. Men take on women's parts and women take on men's parts. Costumes, which do not disguise the performers, often exaggerate the physical qualities of the person being lampooned. A favourite costume is meant to make fun of Malietoa, the current Head of State, whose sexual pursuit of young women is one of the most common subjects of gossip throughout the country. It includes a floral cod-piece of great complexity. Another, impersonating a previous prime-minister who is, even by Samoan standards, a very large man, is so big it often takes two actors to manipulate.

The performances take place on the *malae,* and everyone in the village, as well as people from surrounding villages, attend and join in, calling comments to the performers, adding their own insults and jokes to those levelled at the people being mimicked. The performance space is usually directly in front of the ranking *matai*'s home. They not only attend, but will add comments of their own to insults directed at themselves. In the *fale'aitu*, as Mageo notes in discussing the role of the transvestites [*fa'afafine*] in these performances [1992], the bodies of the actors, if not of all the villagers, are elided, and a geography of play is mapped over the geography of formal roles. The body enacted in the performance becomes a body simulating some other presence, taking the sacred and powerful status of the people depicted, and inverting it, transforming it into play and criticism. Dignity is inverted, the sacredness of the *malae* replaced by the carnality, and even the danger, of the periphery. *Fale'aitu* means, literally, ghost house, which should be more liberally glossed as "the place of the *aitu*," that is the place of discipline and danger, obligation and punishment. For the length of the performance the sacred heart of the village becomes, instead, a space in which danger and asociality are invited and confronted.

Mageo [1992 and especially 1998] suggests the *fale'aitu* gives release to the frustrations of living in a ranked society such as Samoa, and also serve as a way of inscribing the processes of historical transformation on the social conscience of Samoans. From the perspective of embodiment, however, the inversion of work and play, sacredness and carnality, and the safety of the village centre and the danger of the uncivilized periphery, enacts on the bodies participating in these performances, a pervasive and subtle reinforcement of how space is created by the manner in which bodies are deployed. Bodies in the *fale'aitu* become, at least momentarily, some other kind of body, which reminds and re-enacts the experiential distinctions of appropriate space which are integral to Samoan sociality and embodiment. *Fale aitu*, by creating a formal space of masquerade, simulation, and inversion, stand as an exemplary enactment of the vigorous ambiguity of Samoan discipline and transgression.

Sex and Obligation[4]

Working and playing with the body are combined in matters surrounding the appropriate deployment of sexual bodies as well, again within this geography of dignified space. Information about sexual activities is based on personal interviews with close Samoan friends, and on more than 100 detailed sex history interviews conducted with boys, men and, mostly older women. It is reported and discussed here with the full permission of the people who talked to me about these things. It is also, so far as I know, the first systematic attempt to discuss in detail the sexual interests and frameworks of Samoans, something surprising given the most common image of Samoans, fostered by superficial readings of the work of such anthropologists as Margaret Mead, is of a casual and easygoing licentiousness.[5] One hope I have, though not the overriding one, is that what follows goes some distance to correcting and clarifying the ways in which that image is both remarkably accurate and, as remarkably, misguided and misleading.

I must acknowledge, however, that my discussion here, while rigorous, is neither complete nor comprehensive. For one thing, the sites of control and interest in matters related to sex are multiplying, becoming increasingly institutionalized and rationalized, fixing in modes of surveillance and in rigid codes of conduct aspects of embodiment which are also quite fluid and transgressive. This makes the field of sexual activity difficult to map. This becomes even more complicated by certain aspects of the Samoan discourses and practices of propriety.

There is a strong dispreference for younger women to talk with men about many of these matters. This is not a matter of secrecy, or even of modesty, but, as I noted earlier, follows from the dynamic tension in the husband-wife relationship, on the one hand and on the centrality of the brother-sister relationship on the other. All heterosexual relationships in Samoa are indivisible from a singular and all encompassing concern with reproduction, of the family, and thus of the community as a whole. This is perhaps the strongest imperative in all of *Fa'a Samoa* and so cross-sex discussions of sex are never simply about sex. Most of my information on women comes from conversations with older women and as such, adds a different complication, the effect of retrospection. What these women recalled of their lives must not be seen as distorted, however. Rather, in talking about their lives as young girls and young women, they are actually talking about a different version of themselves, one with different objectives, obligations and bodies. The idea that biologically identical persons can yet have completely different bodies is something Duden [1991] demonstrates compellingly in her comparison of 18th and 20th century German women. What I am arguing for here is a similar recognition of the historicity of bodies in individual life courses. It is not simply a matter that ones experience of a fixed body is different at different points in the life course, but that the body is objectively different as well and that it can be related to as something which was me but is not me any longer. The body, as an object through which and because of which subjectivity is instanced, will be a different object depending on the point in history it is encountered, and even, at least in the case of Samoan bodies, depending on the particular context in which it is, at least momentarily, being deployed.

But it cannot be overstated that, not only in my conversations with older women, but with mean as well, I was part of a recollection, a remembered account. In discussing women here, I have restricted myself to generalities precisely because my interests are in what Samoans are doing with their bodies today. The insights I gained from these discussions have helped my understanding, but some other researcher, a woman, will need to follow up on this more fully than I can, even though I feel my grasp of women's sexual lives is sufficiently detailed and thorough. Indeed, as I noted earlier on, the problem of ambiguity and transgression in Samoan gendering and sexing makes it quite reasonable to treat men and women as, in almost all regards, fundamentally the same. However, final problem. As a man, my talking about these things would be insulting to the women who shared their life histories with me. They did so freely, but within the rules of propriety and respect which operate in Samoa, rather than those which may or may not hold in anthropology. I have tried to abide by that confidence, and hope I have not strayed over the line of my Samoan friends welcome and trust. My Samoan informants have an interest in the way they are talked about and in what follows I have been guided by that interest much more than my own academic ones. This aspect of embodiment and social control is of fundamental importance, all the more so as the HIV/AIDS pandemic stands poised to spread throughout the Pacific with a vigour similar to that we have seen in southern Africa in the last decade. Since one of my goals in this book is siting health in the context of embodied analysis, I feel compelled to talk about sex, but I do so with deference, if not necessarily with delicacy.[6]

Foucault [1980 and elsewhere] has argued for seeing the opening up of talk about sex as evidence, not of a release from repression and control, but as a new mode of surveillance and control through discourse. The strong disinclination Samoans show for talking openly about sex, which can easily be read as repression, can also be read, as Mageo [1998] demonstrates clearly, as a ground for loquacious misdirection. She has shown more fully than I propose to do here, that talk about sex in Samoa is actually quite extensive, but is embedded in other discourses about such things as food, *aitu*, mythological histories and so on. Her analysis of sex talk, and of sex work, focuses on cultural systems of meaning and knowledge, and they way these are engaged in constructing a meaningful social self, and so approaches sex from the head outward, if you will. My discussion, on the other hand, approaches sex from the body outward to social field which bodies engage and create. But the importance of sex in Samoan self presentation must not be underestimated.

One of the major points of contention raised by Freeman, in his critique of Mead's work in Samoa, was the portrait of easygoing sexuality, which Mead had described [1983:226-253]. Freeman, and others working in Samoa, have noted that Samoans are often reticent to speak of sexual matters [see, for example, Fitzgerald 1989:40-41 *passim*]. At the same time, most work on Samoa, with the exception of Freeman's, also notes that Samoans are expressive and very sensual in their sexual pursuits [see, for example Shore 1981; Mageo 1992]. I believe the source of this apparent contradiction lies in the presence, in Samoa, of two linked, but separate, modes of sexual practice.[7]

Samoans enact two different kinds of sexual body one related to family and the other to sensuality — *fai'āiga* and *mea lēaga* respectively. These are keyed to their relationship to the levels of dignity which attach to the space and social implications within which sex occurs. At the heart of adult sexuality is *fai'āiga*, the legitimate sexual intercourse of husbands and wives. *Fai'āiga* is "sacred, it is the thing that is about families and making strong and big families," one woman told me.

> It is funny to think about, but it is not a funny thing like what the boys are looking for on the roads at night. No, to do that thing in the house is to be a husband and a wife and not a child anymore playing with their things like that baby there. It is a sacred thing, Douglass, because it tells that story which is about being in a family and making a family for you and for your *'āiga*.

The other, the sensual, play-like sexuality mostly associated with being young is not so closely guarded, though it is subject to as rigorous a set of rules and obligations as the other. But its social peril, though very real, is of a different order.

It is the sexuality of family that Samoans demur from speaking about, and this which makes Samoans look repressed and modest in their erotic life. So much is at stake in this area of sexuality, including not only the commitment made between a husband and wife, but also commitments and obligations to the 'āiga and the community as a whole, that speaking about it is troubling and difficult, not forbidden.[8] It is especially troubling because it combines what Samoans see as one of the most difficult to control appetites of individuals, with the most important aspect of Samoan adult sexuality—making a family by making children. The husband-wife relationship depends, for its success, on the control of loto: those behaviours which are the most resistant to social conditioning, of which sex is the most intransigent. The husband-wife relationship is infused with tension and distress, because sex is vital and actively pursued, and ambiguated by deference and modesty.

This tension collides directly with the brother-sister relationship. As I described in an earlier chapter, the brother-sister relationship is about mutual respect, support and protection. What it is not about is sexual desire. So strong is the prohibition against incest, that Samoans consider marrying anyone with even the furthest cousin relationship to be lēaga [Shore 1981]. However, sex is so deeply engrained in the family space that brothers and sisters are confronted with it daily. Husbands and wives have sex in their homes, at night, surrounded by other sleeping family members. This makes sex a regular and readily observable activity.

At the same time, young men told me how important it was to never appear as a sexual person in front of their sisters, while young women were adamant in their determination that their brothers must never see their sexual parts, because this would invite incest. The result is a combination of tension and deference in this relationship. Joking between brothers and sisters is often brutal and demeaning, sisters calling their brothers dogs and pigs, while brothers joke about such things as their sisters lack of beauty, clumsiness, and rarely and always with immediate apology, about their sexual behaviour. These are jokes of displacement, a repeating pattern of release through which their embodiment as sexual beings, a central aspect of their development through young adulthood into maturity, can be sustained in an environment where the deployment of sexual bodies is closely circumscribed and formalized. At the same time, sister stands iconically for all unmarried women of a young mans generation, such that the waitress in a nightclub is referred to, generically, as sister. In a sense, all young unmarried women are both potential wives and potential sisters at the same time, a contradiction which I think energizes the brother-sister dyad, while at the same time making it profoundly troubling and troublesome.

Husbands and wives, the most intimate dyadic relationship for Samoans, are quiet and respectful toward each other, in comparison to this often brutal and antagonistic engagement between brothers and sisters. So solemn are the connections between husbands' and wives' bodies that they themselves, while willing to talk in detail about sex in general, will refuse politely to speak of their own bodily connections. So formal, constrained, and important is the embodiment of family in *fai'āiga,* that, while sexual joking about others forms a key idiom in conversations between sex segregated groups of men and women, even the slightest allusion to a member of the group's sexual relations with his or her wife or husband can lead to enmity, which may last years, and in at least two cases of which I am aware, to murder.

Where *fai'āiga* is a source of concern and embarrassment, *ta'alo* [literally, play or fun], is a mode of casual sexuality which is both approved and encouraged, and is often the subject of jokes and playful insults. Play in this sense is the pursuit of illicit sex, the one sanctioned space for individualized bodies in the Samoan social field. It is in this distinction that the core of Freeman's attack on Mead, in which he argues that Mead was misled by her informants, evaporates [1983:240, 289-90]. It is not, I suggest, that Mead's informants duped her, while Freeman's older female informants told him the truth. Rather, because sex, sexuality, and sexual morality, are tied to the constitution of status, dignity, and appropriate space, among so many other things which vary over the life course, both sets of informants, and even the same informants at different times in their life if Freeman [1999] is to be believed were telling the truth. However, it was a truth which was contingent and changeable because it was a truth about two different thing. If the experience of the body in Samoa is ineluctably connected with such culturing issues as the meanings of space, and the pursuit of dignity, as I have been arguing here, then the apparently contradictory assertions of these informants makes simple, cultural sense. They were telling the truth about two different bodies, two different people.[9]

This problem of multiple sexualized bodies in Samoa combines with a range of other complications in the enactment and constraint of sexual behaviour, some conceptual and some structural, which the next two charts illustrate. These complications apply in equal force, however, to all matters of order and social control and obligation in Samoa.

The first complication is a generic one and relates to the question of what Herdt has called sexual cultures [1997, 1999]. Sex is enacted inside a web of differentially weighted conditioning factors, such as culture, psychology, systems of morality and modesty, power and reproductive control, and of course gender, and where it exists, sexuality. In Samoa, as elsewhere, this is further complicated by life course changes which can effectively transform or at least re-rank the salience of any of these as components of the sexual culture or cultures any individual participates in or is constrained by. The effect, I suggest, is to make sex much more inscrutable than it is often described. Without assuming, for example, that sex and identity are indivisibly linked, which most analysis of sexual behaviour assumes to be true, because sexual acts are always connected with issues of reproduction and, especially, social reproduction, it is safe to assume that sex is always engaged in processes of self consciousness, even if they are not the interior mental processes of psychological approaches to sex and sexuality. Sex can be read for many things, from nationalism [Parker, Sommer, and Yaeger 1991] to the epidemiology of pandemic disease [Herdt 1997]. And all through this, the sexual life of the individual is shifting, reorienting, and reconfiguring itself as his or her body is watched, touched, moved and manipulated.

Figure 7.3 illustrates this concatenation of interests and attentions as they are engaged in the sexually active body. Of particular importance are those things which go without saying, those aspects of embodied experience which have been completely naturalized by socialization and praxis. Desire and arousal, embarrassment and bravado, guilt and ecstasy are all inscribed in a special code of experience which is fetishized into thoughtlessness. These are things which just happen, which are just part of being human. That they are, ontologically, particular encultured figurations of observation and social control is elided by their experience as mechanical and cellular. This makes sexuality in its various ramifications a central site of social control, and I suggest this is true in all cultures wherever they might be located on a scale of explicit repression. In the case of Samoa, my informants talked about the complications of sex with a resignation consistent with their experience of these conditions as "just the way things are." This encultured resignation also means that sexuality can be engaged as a primary site of transformations in social control, either in terms of controlling structures or, more fundamentally, in terms of underlying conceptual frames which control structures enact. In my conversations with many young Samoan men, it was apparent there was a sense of dissonance between an experience of gender and sexing which was flexible, ambiguous and manipulable, and a different, competing articulation in which gender and sex were coming to be experienced as objective and static, governed by fixed moral categories which transcended context. This fixing of sex and gender is manifesting itself in different ways, such as in the emergence of an identity based homosexuality, or in changes in the patterns of spouse to spouse violence, which is increasingly victimizing women.

In the context of inherently complicated conditioning components of sex, Samoans have to manouver around the competing and conflicting obligations of various institutions and structures which enact and enforce social order and propriety. Referring back to Figure 7.1, it is possible to see how this network conditions sexuality and sexual behaviour. Each authoritative and obligating site in this system, has an interest in the sexual body, whether it is a familial interest, a moral one, some economic inter-

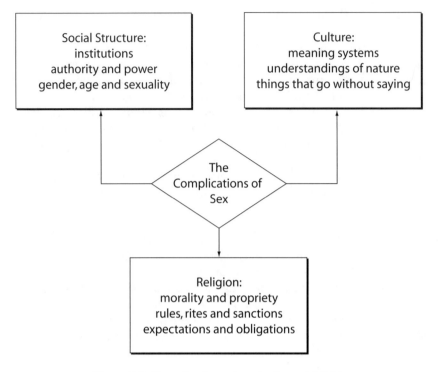

Figure 7.3 Complications of sex in the social field.

est, or those interests connected to peer relations or to proscriptive relations such as the brother-sister dyad. In each instance, these structures and institutions are present, as very real actors, in the enactment of sexual behaviour such that, not only does sex in Samoa often not take place in exclusive privacy, the presence of these interests arrayed in the social field ensures that sexual partners never are, in fact or experience, actually alone. Each sex act, each sexual thought is constrained by status and age distinctions, courtship interest and obligations, and the important and conditional proscriptions of maturing into full members of the community. At the same time there are sensual interests, whether erotic or ludic, and important considerations of identity and self-conception. At the same time sex talk, that is, who can speak and who can be spoken to or with, about what, when and to what purpose, further complicate the landscape of connections within which embodiment and sex are enacted. Within this field of multiple engagements, Samoan sexual life is played out from childhood onward.

Children are expected, though not openly encouraged, to engage in sexual play. Masturbation by boys is not discouraged until late adolescence, when most people feel that boys should have found more appropriate sexual outlets. Nevertheless, it is not allowed in public from even the earliest years of childhood. A boy caught masturbating will not be told to stop, however. Instead, he will be told to "go into the banana patch" or "go behind the cook-house," spaces of relative invisibility. From the earliest moments of sexual exploration, boys enact in their sensual play an emerging sense of appropriate space, and of the obligations surveillance imposes on behaviour.

Sexual exploration, and sexual education flourish in adolescence. Average age of first heterosexual intercourse for boys is around 13 and for girls, around 16. As well, by age 6 or seven most boys will have formed a particularly special relationship referred to as either *soa* or *pa'aga*, a close and intimate partner who shares circumcision, tattooing, and sexual education.[10] The importance of this relationship for men cannot be overstated. There are four fundamental relationships: parent-child, and *matai-'āiga*, which are mimetic extensions of each other, the first private and the second public, and husband-wife and brother-sister, which are inversions of each other. The first is sexualized and complementary and the second, anerotic and often antagonistic. The *soa* partnership combines features of all four in the complex of activities *soa* partners pursue together. *Soa* is a generic word for a special kind of relationship in which one person acts on behalf of another, something Mageo transcribes as "go-between." That is, the *soa* partner acts as an agent on someone's behalf. In this adolescent version of this kind of partnership, boys explore and experience all aspects of deference, sharing, support, and authority, enacting in the intimate relationships of their youth, all the kinds of bodies they will be and encounter throughout their lives. Their *soa* relationship incorporates partnership, mutuality, and the body together in a web of activities and implications for which there is no North American equivalent.

There is no conventional prohibition against casual homosexual sex among young men in Samoa, although attitudes which moralize homosexuality have certainly been adopted by some Christian Samoans. However, these religious restrictions are applied almost exclusively to adult homosexuals, when they are applied at all. Recent discussions with some informants in Samoa lead me to believe that homosexuality, as a moral category, is gaining ground in Samoa. I have received several reports of violence against *fa'afafine* in the last year or so, in which the attackers, always a group of young men, called the victim "fag" or "queer." At the same time, there is an emergent sense of homosexual identity, as something both life long and distinctive from some other male identity, among many of my informants, both those who are presently *fa'afafine* and those who are not. How widespread this phenomenon is is difficult to measure from afar, and impossible to discern from such scattered reports of violence and so on. However, it is consistent with my argument here that configurations of practice, enacted bodies, and self-concept are always changing in Samoa. Like the adoption of "traditional" tattoos as a badge of nationalism rather than as a marker of obligation to a chief, the emergence of a more fixed set of sexualities in Samoa is part of the ongoing process of accommodation and transgression which characterizes so much of Samoan social life.

It is generally expected that boys will have some homosexual experience in their adolescence and *soa* partners can also be sexual partners, though not in any romantic sense. This is play more than anything else, a play which teaches, but play nonetheless. Punning on the word *soa* can be quite ribald, and draws upon associations with the authority and deference structures, expressing the conventionalized, and generally positive nature of these relationships. A boy may refer to his partner as *sua*, meaning a vessel for holding liquid, an unabashed reference to fellatio or mutual masturbation, or, *sua*², which means the special food prepared for and presented to a *matai* at important functions. While the sex, when it occurs, between *soa* needs to be understood as *ta'alo* [play], it is also an important form of support and generosity. The punning on *sua*² incorporates this aspect of the *soa* relationship quite tellingly. Such partnerships also incorporate the mutuality of deference and support because the sexual relationship between *soa* partners, like the relationship of partnership in tattooing and circumcision, is not unilateral, but about mutual presence in each other's actions.

This is a neccessarily idealized explanation of this core relationship. Key here is the issue of mutuality and support in body-making experiences. In particular, the possibility of a sexual aspect of this relationship is difficult to capture adequately in so brief a description because of the complicated implications of the distinction between young peoples sexual play and other forms of sexual activity. And so the issue of sexual acts between *soa* partners needs to be understand as a facet of this relationship and not a central feature of it. At the same time, these observations are consistent with Mead's observations about the absence of a generic prohibitions against homosexual activity. Where it departs from Mead's comments is in recognizing that the lack of a prohibition does not mean a lack of often quite complex and rigid rules, rules which are governed by the kinds of bodies we have at different points in our lives.

Boys are also expected to have considerable heterosexual experience. This is seen as a way of learning about sex, rather than courtship per se. The pursuit of heterosexual partners by adolescent boys and young men is play and fun and a way of mapping out relations of desire and obligation. However, while the foregoing sounds idyllic and liberated, it is tied inexorably to the fundamental geography of space and dignity.

Ta'alo, that is, sexual play in all of its rambunctious forms, is relegated to the undignified and asocial space of plantations and gardens and even, for the brave at least, to the *aitu* occupied bush. This circumscribes sexual behaviour as rigorously as repressions in more articulately regulatory societies, but it does so through a different mechanism, that of creating kinds of space through what bodies do in them.[11] You can see this mapping of restriction in the flow of semen as it relates to different sites of dignified space in Samoa. As I noted in Chapter 4, Samoans do not have a formal and restrictive semen distribution complex such as that found in some areas of Papua New Guinea. Semen, for Samoans, is meant to circulate and be distributed, rather than hoarded and recycled. Indeed, a distinction between extensive and restrictive semen distribution appears to be one of the distinguishing features in comparing Melanesian and Polynesian societies. However, like in sexual matters, the absence of repressive restrictions does not mean there are no restrictions at all.

The extent and path of semen distribution is determined by the nature of the space in which it is used. Within the village and the family circle, semen is closely restricted. It must circulate, and is expected to circulate often, but only along a path between husband and wife. Beyond the village however, semen circulates in multiple paths, between close male friends, between boys and girls who form many serially monogamous sexual relationships, and between the boy and his own body, in the form of masturbation, where he demonstrates his potency and the proper volume of his semen in an act of both physical and self gratification. This is not to suggest, however, that promiscuity is random, although it is at times quite casual. At the same time that boys are circulating their semen in casual sex, they are calculating and enacting embodied relationships between themselves and the girls, some of whom may be potential wives. As one boy put it, "I leave my semen in many villages, but there are some where it cannot go and I know this. Those are the villages where I might have sisters or where I should find a wife." Incest prohibitions, and concern over behaving sexually in front of a "sister" extend to choice of casual heterosexual partners because in their pursuit of sexual victories [and the boys I interviewed saw this as winning something from the girl], they are also pursuing and inscribing, in very intimate ways, the rules and relationships of kinship, choosing partners with only apparent nonchalance since there is, in even the most apparently casual of sexual partner choices, close attention to kin prohibitions. Ironically, the effect of this is make closely related women the prime choice of casual sexual partner, since they are not suitable as wives because of their kin proximity. A wife, like a husband, must be as distantly related as possible. The effect of this is to bring sexual play, sexual learning, and casual sexuality closest to the young man or young woman's household itself, adding tension and deep ambiguity to the sexual aspects of the household space, and in particular, to the intricacies of the brother-sister relationship. As one young man put it too me, "here we marry our cousins, but we have sex with our sisters."

A striking application of gendered distinctions emerges out of conversations with older adults about the sexual behavior of the young. Boys are, as I have indicated, expected to be relatively promiscuous during the adolescence and early adulthood. This is boys being *ta'a*, roaming and exploring, in a manner similar to animals and is seen as part of their path from incomplete and animal like creature to full human status which arrives with adulthood and marriage. I would even go so far as to suggest that a Samoan is not fully human until he or she has married and begun a new family by having children. In contrast, girls who are promiscuous in adolescence and young adulthood were more often referred to as *paumutu*, which most dictionaries gloss as promiscuous. However, this is a word reserved almost exclusively for girls, and in my discussions and conversations was applied to boys sarcastically. Pressed on what people meant by this word, they would speak of how promiscuous girls were nothing more than receptacles for boys penises, or, were abrogating their responsibility to their families by being capricious rather than sufficiently calculating in their courtship. Samoan speech is remarkably figurative and *paumutu* with its allusions to broken vessels, the bodily connections of kinship, and submission to authority exemplifies this metaphorical richness. But within this richness a gendered coding of obligation in courtship appears to be operating which suggests that within the ambiguation and transgressive practices of sexuality in Samoa, a more fixed set of tensions exist. This play of fixity and transience, of ambiguity and perspicuity, is key to the energizing effect embodiment and experience have on the enactment of culture and the world.

In my discussions with friends and informants, I encountered many restrictions on specific sex acts, although there are few restrictions on sex itself, at least for adolescents.[12] Most of the restrictions they spoke of involved male to male relations and referred to such things as the posture of the participants during sex, particularly avoiding positions which mimic the sexual posture of men and women. There are also restrictions on certain acts, such as fellatio, which many said should only be performed at night, while mutual masturbation between males can take place during the day. Finally, male to male body to body rubbing [*frottage*], was felt to feminize both participants, because it mimics heterosexual intercourse, and so is avoided. The frequency of either heterosexual or homosexual acts is not restricted, and there are no restrictions related to menstruation or any ritual or spiritual restrictions. Semen which is discharged on the skin should be washed off because its properties of triggering the growth of tissue could cause growths to develop on the skin. There is no restriction on consuming semen, but no special value is attached to it. Some sex acts are also restricted by age. For example, fellatio and cunnilingus are considered inappropriate for older men and women, but not for moral reasons. Many people explained to me that the posture required to perform these acts puts one participant, who is, generically at least, ranked equal by virtue of age and assumed accomplishment, in a position of servility in relation to the body of another, which would be considered inappropriate and embarrassing. Finally, certain sex acts and positions are preferred over others, and without lapsing completely into prurience here, the preference appears to be governed by a concern for mutuality of pleasure, on the one hand, and a strong desire to be able to observe the face of ones partner and to avoid observing the genitals.

A different complication relates to sex acts between men and *fa'afafine*. *Fa'afafine* are physically males, as I noted earlier, but they and their bodies are not conceptually male or female. They are something distinctive, a third transient sex. I say transient because *fa'afafine*, for the most part, become male by their late 20's or early 30's, marrying, and fathering children. Many informants noted, however, that in recent years more and more *fa'afafine* are sustaining their *fa'afafine* status into middle age and beyond. However, what is distinctive about sex with *fa'afafine*, beyond the fact it cannot be called homosexual, whatever the sex of the other partner, is that it is prohibited *in the village*, but is not prohibited in and of itself. The *fa'afafine* is the legitimate sex partner of young men learning about sex, and in some ways the *fa'afafine* allows young males to learn about appropriate sexual relations with women since only *fa'afafine* should engage in passive anal sex. Many young Samoan men described this aspect of their relationships with *fa'afafine* as "learning to be with a woman." The *fa'afafine*, as a woman-like substitute, avoids some of the dangers and problems of determining incest relations because there is no kinship prohibition on sex between young men and *fa'afafine*. The *fa'afafine* exemplifies a kind of embodying strategy, where the apparent substance of the body is elided by its enactment, becoming some other body, whatever the apparent similarity between males and *fa'afafine* physically. That this ambiguation of morphology is relegated to the dark periphery should not be surprising, because not only is it an aspect of the fundamental ambiguities of gender and sexuality in Samoa, it is also not easily reconciled with the de-sexed, but persistently sexual space of the household, where the *fa'afafine*'s ambiguous sexual nature contradicts the restraint and decorum of the household as a sexual space. *Fa'afafine* are not excluded from any village affairs, can at least theoretically become *matai*, and participate in all family and village discussions and decisions. However, it is possible, as Besnier [1994:560 n47] has noted, to over-romanticize the positive position of the *fa'afafine* in Samoan society. The recent effort by Mageo

[1992] to disentangle a history of the role and meaning of the *fa'afafine* is interesting but also somewhat disappointing because the *fa'afafine* is conceived, in her argument, solely in terms of what the *fa'afafine* means to Samoan males and females. *Fa'afafine* are transformed into a strategy employed by some other, more real, sex, which elides the erotics and phenomenology of *fa'afafines* own experiences and embodying practices. At the same time, to paint the *fa'afafine* as an always positive member of the community ignores the very real tension in the *fa'afafine's* position as a butt of jokes, as a disposable sexual outlet and as an object of occasional, and increasing, violence and brutality. I am primarily interested here in the *fa'afafine's* penis and semen, because they look and behave the same way as men's, but are not, conceptually or practically, male genitals. Unravelling the nature and role of all genders in Samoa is beyond the scope of what I am describing here. It is an issue which has been inadequately dealt with in the literature on either Samoa or on gender in Polynesia, a situation improved only somewhat by the publication of a volume of papers on third genders [Herdt 1994]. It is also an issue which I am exploring, in ongoing work on *fa'afafine* and their experiences in Samoa. As I am sure is now apparent from their repeated appearances in these pages, the *fa'afafine* are an inescapable conundrum in understanding Samoan embodiment. That conundrum speaks to the complex heart of Samoan discipline and its connections and disconnections with gendering and sex. I discussed briefly *fa'afine* and the problem of the encroachment of rigid modes of body experience in Chapter 2, and want to simply stress that the *fa'afine* is a fundamental analytic problem in understanding *Fa'a Samoa*.

The enforcement of codes of sexuality as a process of social control needs to be understood not only in the larger strictures of moral systems, but in the minutiae of intimate application, as these examples suggest. But something worth stressing is the fact, borne out by my conversations about sex acts not only with Samoans but with young men working in the commercial sex trade in Canada, and with gay men living in and around a gay neighbourhood in Toronto, Canada, is that these minute practical expressions of sexual prescription, because of the intimacy of the site at which they are interpreted and enacted, are perhaps the most subjective aspect of the experience of sex as a modality of social surveillance and control. That tiny variations in posture, timing, or location can fundamentally alter the controlling effects of sex systems illustrates how powerful and complex sex is as a system of managing embodied experience. The sexual body is a strategy of embodiment and a strategic engagement with the physical and cultural world, that is, a strategy in which body, space, and culture conjoin in creating each other.

Making sense of the deployment of bodies is central to making a model of embodiment sensible and comprehensive. What needs to be taken into account are the connections which are enacted between appetites, obligations, privacy and selfishness. In Samoa, play and work are two such sites at which these issues are enacted in the constitution of meaningful bodies engaged as strategic dispositions. Through these enactments, bodies and space, along with values, principles, and expectations, become coterminous, whether in the body returning from the plantation, or lying with its girl-friend under a palm tree in the crepuscular midnight of a South Pacific full moon, or pushing a rickety wooden "truck" along a lonely dirt road, singing.

In discussing the disciplines of play and work, and of sex and sexual behaviour, I am arguing that even the most mundane of acts of pleasure are an inextricably tangled skein of meaning, and the creation of meaning. What I am also arguing is that what is being enacted on, with, and by the body, is always about discipline. Even in the darkness of the periphery, control and observation are being enacted on, and by the bodies which are deployed and engaged there. Through the bodies in the dark, the dignity of the centre encompasses all social space. The virtue of the temple and the forum collide and collude with the pleasures of the sauna.

Chapter 8

Bodies of Danger/Bodies Endangered: Illness, Healing, and the Pursuits of Dignity

I assert that "disease" does not exist. It is therefore illusory to think that one can "develop beliefs" about it or "respond" to it. What does exist is not disease, but practices.

> Francois Delaporte
> Disease and Civilisation

"What are you going through," is all you need to ask.

> Simone Weil

Pita lay on the sleeping mat, rocking restlessly in his sleep. Occasionally he would moan softly, and his mother would reach over and wipe away the sweat on his face with the edge of her *lavalava*, now stained from several hours of this constant duty. Around the mat were his two brothers, an aunt, the wife of the Methodist minister, and a Samoan healer, who sat holding a bible in one hand, and a bundle of bright green leaves in the other. Every several minutes she would take the leaves and rub them over Pita's stomach, reciting a portion of the Christian Lord's Prayer, in English, as she did. Then she would sit back on her heels and bow her head, praying silently.

The day before, Pita had been walking along the main road of the village of Vaimoso, on his way home from buying his mother some tea bags at the local village store. A loud blast of thunder over the mountains startled him, and he turned suddenly to look in the direction where the storm was gathering strength as it passed over the island. In turning he fell, knocking his head with a harsh impact on a recently fallen coconut. He had lain there, no one knew for how long, until a man and his children, coming along the road, found him and carried him home to his small green house in the banana patch behind where I lived. Through the storm darkened gloom I saw the group coming along the road, could hear them talking in hushed tones, but barely paid attention, turning back to my computer screen and the transcription of an interview I had completed earlier that day with a man about to leave for New Zealand for heart surgery. I managed to finish one more paragraph before Charlie, Pita's brother, was suddenly outside my window, breathless, asking if I would drive him to a nearby village to bring back a *fofō* because Pita was dying, he was being killed by an *aitu* and Mafo'e, Pita and Charlie's mother, could think of no way to stop it from happening.

Injury, like illness, is not simply something which occurs. They require explanation, because they engage the frailty of the enacted body, and render opaque the connected practices of embodiment which conjoin consciousness, cultural, and the lived sensory experience of our bodies. Questions of discipline and punishment, propriety and appropriate presence, and the multiple lines that connect the complexes of good and bad, are important processes where the body is understood and enacted. With illness and injury, perhaps, the greatest work of embodiment is carried out, because it is in illness and injury that everything the body is, and does, is directly threatened and undermined. The sick body is a body at the heart of the dissolution of the very world that the body has created.[1]

In this chapter I will explore some of the ground on which illness is recognized and dealt with, as one of the key instantiations of the Samoan geography of embodiment. Much of what I understand about the Samoan body, in both health and illness, comes from months spent talking with traditional healers, and most importantly, their patients; from the diagnostic events I personally witnessed, and from illness event interviews in which informants were asked to recount the progress of an illness they had experienced in the year previous.[2] It was in this participation, and in the regular and wide ranging conversations about illness that my still incomplete understanding of the Samoan body began to emerge. I cannot stress the importance, in particular, of everyday conversations about illness in Samoa too strongly. Talking about illness and healing is the one are where Samoans talk freely, indeed almost constantly, about their bodies. Samoan everyday talk seems drawn to illness and healing as a discursive space where they can talk fully and openly about the tensions and ambiguities of their embodied praxis. This talk, which monitors bodies in the community, also deflects and disguises dangerous bodies through dissembling and inventive misdirection, issues I return to in the concluding chapter. What follows here is an outline of the Samoan practice of health as it implicates the persistent concerns with dignity, humility and strength which underlie all aspects of Samoan embodiment.

I will frame my discussion within the context of a Samoan model of illness events [Figure 8.1] as well as Samoans experiences of the qualities and characteristics of their anatomy and biology.[3] I am not contrasting this biology to some other, more accurate, biology, however. The biological model Samoans have is neither less nor more accurate in terms of its reli-

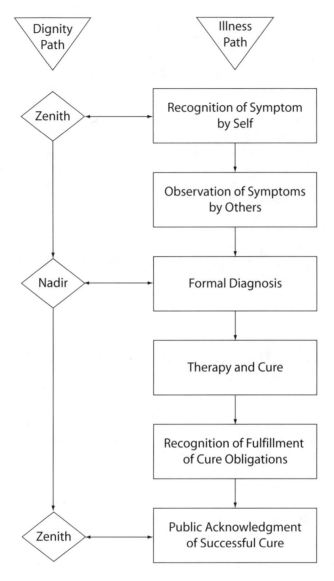

Figure 8.1 The path of illness in Samoa.

ability than the model we, as Westernised bodies, apply to our own experiences. However, Samoans have, as a result of their experiences and understandings of their bodies, different organs than what might be found, for example, in the bodies of North Americans. In the study of embodiment, biology needs to be approached from the point of view of these models, and not solely from the perspective of scientific anatomy. More important than what the body is as an organic object, the body needs to be understood as being "what we do with it," as well.[4]

A critical model of embodiment must avoid the pitfall of contrasting social and biological realities [Scheper-Hughes and Lock 1987]. This approach, as I discussed in Chapter 2, dominates much of medical anthropology. The risk such an approach takes lies in leaving implicit the subtle, evaluative aspect of these comparisons. Local biologies are often implicitly measured against scientific biology in terms of accuracy, reliability, and validity. While such approaches can provide important insights into health practice, as well as helping to explore how the introduction of new models of anatomy are adapted by local communities [see, for example, Frankel 1989], what is lost in such analyses is the effect of local understandings on the lived experience of the body itself.

At the same time, a model of embodiment needs to explode the clinical encounter analytically, in order to deconstruct not only how the body is manipulated in illness, but also how expertise itself is constituted. It needs to clarify the relationship between expert models and other body cultures which may co-exist in a given society, through a more thorough ethnographic account of the notion of expertise itself.[5]

What Every\body Knows:
Samoan Expertise as Action

Jordan suggests that "for any particular domain several knowledge systems exist, some of which, by consensus, come to carry more weight than others, either because they explain the state of the world better for the purposes at hand [efficacy] or because they are association with a stronger power base [structural superiority] and usually both" [1997:56]. This generalizing observation, while focussed as Jordan is, on childbirth practices, leaves the whole notion of what exactly constitutes expertise under-theorized and under-nourished. Because she focuses on something as amorphous as "knowledge systems" which are, after all, analytic abstractions derived from the models we use as anthropologists to codify the worlds we study, the ongoing nature of expert systems as social processes is lost. This is a common analytic problem, a kind of taking the rhetoric of the expert class at its word, and reflects our own subservience to the primacy of scholarly traditions as knowledge systems. While competing knowledge systems may well be effects of power and legitimation, as Jordan goes on to argue, that can never be assumed. This is an error I was guilty of for quite some time during the early part of my initial fieldwork in Samoa. I sought out healers, and peppered them with questions about models and practices like some supplicant at the feet of a holy teacher. It was only later, after my own illnesses, and after the illnesses of my Samoan family and friends, that I can to see that expertise, the entire medical knowledge system in Samoa, was not a matter of experts but of doing, ability, success.

In Samoa, expertise is about skill and not solely about knowledge. That is, the healer [fofō], like the tufuga [tattooist/circumciser] and the matai themselves, are expert by virtue of the skill they bring to bear on their tasks. But the knowledge of illness meaning and curing practices is general knowledge, shared by everyone. The healer recognized and respected solely by skill and past success. As such, no one is a medical expert in Samoa in our sense of having specialist knowledge. Instead, the expert is the most successful at applying this knowledge, and not simply the most knowledgeable person, a distinction which needs to be borne in mind when thinking about clinical relations in Samoa [Moyle 1974:158; Koskinen 1968:11-12]. Like the matai, whose knowledge of the fa'alupega is secondary to his manipulation and re-representations of that knowledge to the advantage of his 'āiga, the fofō is not a repository of secret knowledge, but a history of the most skilful applications of what is instead common knowledge in actual clinical experience. All participants in the clinical encounter in Samoa are presumed to have the same basic information, but different levels of skill. This, I feel, is a key issue in understanding how Samoans enact illness, because experts do not dominate the process of defining an illness into existence. Rather, expert and patient collude in the process of making symptoms meaningful, and drawing the meaning of the illness from the evidence of the world around them. More importantly, from the perspective of illness as an embodying practice, the generalness of this knowledge, and the importance of consensus and broad participation in the illness defining process, opens illness events up to many forms of manipulation.

An ethnography of the body needs to account, not only for illness events, but also for the overall process of living within, and watching, the body with which illness occurs. It needs to address the fact that the body is a lived experience, of which illness is only one facet, and that illness and health are part of an ongoing, constant process of observation and accounting. Few areas of the practiced body offer complete access to this process of enactment, through which body, being, and experience are conjoined. Desire is one, punishment another, and illness yet another. Kirmayer captures the issue of how illness enjoins us to focus on the multiple aspects of the lived ground of embodiment when he suggests we "[c]ompare: [1] feeling sick; [2] being treated as sick by others; [3] being told you are sick by a doctor; [4] finding your temperature elevated on a thermometer" [1992:324]. My focus here is on how being sick, and the lived enactment of the body in its other aspects, are inseparable and ongoing.[6]

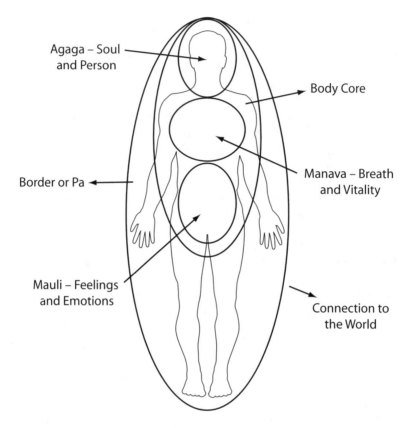

Agaga – Soul and Person

Body Core

Border or Pa

Manava – Breath and Vitality

Mauli – Feelings and Emotions

Connection to the World

Figure 8.2 Body Segments

Samoan Anatomy: Bodies as Motion

I have been arguing throughout this text that the body needs to be understood as a potential for meaning, a potential which is realized through enactment. Anatomy needs to be understood, therefore, not only in the scientific-classificatory-clinical sense, but also as a practice through which the structures and processes of the body are enacted into meaningful existence in daily life. In describing Samoan anatomy then, I am not contrasting folk theories against some truer biological model, in the form, for example, of assertions like "Samoans believe the heart digests food." Rather, in what follows I am adopting a different posture, one which takes Samoans at their word, and accepts that for these people in this place at this time, the heart is a part of the digestive system, and the lungs are water filters.

Samoans divide the body into three components: the interior, the boundary, and things outside, but connected to, the body. Each of these aspects of the body stands in a relationship of interconnectedness and indivisibility with the others, such that the core of the body and the environment of physical and social relationships which encompass the body are part of a single organic unity. That organic unity is not simply the connection of the body with the world, but a technique for embodying the world in which issues of core and outside, process and flow which function at the level of biology are also expressed in such things as the moral geography of villages, or in the enactment of authority and power in the *fono* and *'ava* ceremonies. Like villages, these bodily sites decrease in dignity and sacredness the further one moves from the core. Like villages, the danger of illness is most perilous in its effects on the interior of the body, and like villages the most dangerous site, the place of greatest peril, is the surface of the body where it connects and extends into the rest of the physical world. Figure 8.2 illustrates this dividing up of the body and its connections to the world.

There is an element of ambiguity about the borders between the peripheral organs and limbs or *pā* [boundary or border] and the world around it, which is separate, but connected to the body as part of the body process. As well, these body spaces need to be understood not only as locations, but as sets of relationships between different organic aspects of the body. They enact relationships of connection, flow, and motion rather than simply serving as places where body parts and body processes occur. While I will not discuss the issue of *mana*, the trans-Polynesian concept of energizing power or efficacy [see Keesing 1984; Shore 1989], this is because, in general, this concept was rarely brought up in my conversations with Samoans. However, as Shore notes [1989:138], *mana* needs to be understood in relation to the Polynesian dispreference for defining things in terms of essential qualities and characteristics. *Mana*, therefore, is a state of energy, rather than an energy itself, and in Samoan anatomy is reflected in the properly mapped body standing in a state of healthful readiness to act. The Samoan word for readiness or "ability" [and also for beautiful], *manaia* translates as "being energetic" rather than as "having energy." The healthy body is a condition of *mana* and a fluid state of readiness.

Internal organs, both in the central and peripheral sites of the body, have two collateral qualities which define them as good and proper: location and process. The geography of the internal organs is a key component in the body's proper functioning. Organs have a proper location. Organs also have the tendency to move, or to be shifted, from their proper place, and this is a common cause of illness. Organs do not move wilfully, however. Instead, they are moved by either physical activity or by the interference of *aitu,* who can kick organs out of location or who may actually enter the body and physically move organs about.[7]

Process, the other quality, relates to how organs are connected in the movement of substances or forces throughout the body. All organs are implicated in the flow of body substances, such as food, blood, water, air, faeces, semen or bile. Organs are experienced as conduits through which substances move, the organ in some instances, such as the liver, effecting some change in the substance by adding to it or taking something from it, and in other instances, such as the testicles, serving a muscular function which causes the expulsion of semen in ejaculation.

In general, Samoans have the same organs as those we would recognize, but with important differences. The most obvious is the fact organs move in the viscera, which means the liver can actually end up in a part of the body where we would be unlikely to look for it. Another important difference is the linking of organs into single units. The heart and lungs [*fatu*, a polite word for blood, and *māmā*, the formal word for lungs], for example, are connected as one single multi-component organ, rather than two distinct organs, in the organ/space referred to as the *manava* [breath and stillness]. The heart forces blood in and out of the lungs where it is moistened through breathing, and also settled to avoid its becoming too hot and agitated. Paths between organs are also distinctive. The *manava* is linked directly to the stomach, through which food, blood, and air are conjoined in the stomach's food storing process.

A final difference is the presence of organs which are not found in our own bodies. The most important is the *to'ala*, an ambiguously defined muscular organ which serves as a conduit for energy throughout the viscera, and which is normally located just below the sternum, in a healthy person. The *to'ala* is the most troublesome organ for Samoans because of its tendency to shift position very readily, causing strangulation or blockage of other organs including the blocking of the *fa'aautagata* [womb place], which can result in either barrenness, difficulty in delivery, or deformity of the foetus through pressure or other distortions. The *to'ala* is the most common target of *aitu* attacks on the organs and, I was told, has the potential of actually being expelled from the body accidentally.

In speaking of their bodies, my advisors and informants would often speak in terms of the movement of substances through the body. A good and healthy body is full of all the common substances we recognize, such as urine, blood, bile, and saliva. To be healthy, these substances need to be in constant flow throughout, and then, out of the body. This steady stream of body fluids is an important diagnostic feature of illness recognition, and it also defines for Samoans a manner of movement in the world which recognizes that things enter the body and must leave it in good time and in appropriate volumes. The qualities of these substances as they leave the body are scrutinized for their relative health. For example, faeces should flow easily and should have a soft, though not watery consistency. Menstrual blood,

I was told, should be very bright red, and not black or discoloured. Saliva and semen are related fluids, and should be ample and have a gum-like consistency when exposed to air.

Illness substances such as pus or other discharges from wounds or sores, vomit, bile, and diarrhoea, are understood as a means of ridding the body of unnecessary or foreign substances which impair the internal organ's function. This process of ridding the body may be in the form of excess male or female body part substances, which each sex needs in only limited quantities. It may also be excess in other substances such as water or certain kinds of food, which again the body needs only in restricted quantities. The manifestation of these substances may be the result of a back-up in the flow of substances through appropriate channels in the body, causing them to flow either backwards, as in vomit, or to flow explosively when finally released, as in extreme cases of diarrhoea. Finally, these substances may be foreign matter hazardous to the body, which the body incorporates into other substances and then expels.

The anatomy of the body, then, is experienced and understood by my informants in terms of ranked sites within and around the body, and of the steady flow of substances into, through and out of the body. As such, the body and the village and the world itself as mimetic of each other. Each have a sacred core, where the most important processes of organic life occur. Each also have a functional ring of connection through which the body is tied to, and makes use of, the world around it. Body processes, whether digestion or pregnancy or the creation and expulsion of phlegm, mirror activities and conditions of dignity in the moral ordering of the village, where work and labour sustains the sacred core of both the body and the village, and where the dangerous and undignified detritus of this sustenance are moved out of, and way, from the dignity of both. In experiencing their bodies, Samoans experience, in miniature, the fundamental principles of their socialized universe. In experiencing their material world, they write outward from their bodies a model of order and power.

Symptoms and Signals: Reading the Body for Danger

Symptoms, in Samoa, are both evidence of improper functioning, and signs the body is healthy and proper. While it is possible to distinguish between signs of distress and signs of propriety, it is important to be aware that Samoans do not only attend to their bodies when there is trouble. They are attentive, watchful, and alert, not only to signs of danger, but also to signs of propriety and appropriate function.

There are two issues which need to be raised at the outset. The first relates to the Samoan word *ma'i* which is normally translated as illness. *Ma'i* encompasses everything from cancer to anger to drunkenness to not attending church to paranoid schizophrenia to spirit possession. The English word cannot cover all these conditions and behaviours, and so, using illness to translate *ma'i* requires we qualify ill to mean "in the Samoan sense of some disturbance in proper behaviour, body function, or social relations."

That is the first problem in approaching Samoan illness and symptomatics. The other is in distinguishing symptoms from causes. In what follows I will be talking about body signs as "meaning" illness. This is a convenience rather than an analytic posture on my part, because symptom and cause are often conflated in Samoan illness practice. To questions about whether anger causes illness, is a symptom, or is caused by illness, the most common answers I got was "whose illness" or "which time would that anger have happened." Anger is both a cause and effect of illness, depending on the circumstances and the type of illness. As Albert once put it to me, half joking because he always accused me of taking my questions much too seriously, "you ask if sadness can make me sick. I have to ask you what day of the week was that sadness I had, and maybe what time was it, and then I have to ask who was I sitting with, and maybe I would just ask if you had asked me for my last Vailima [the local beer], and I gave it to you when I was thirsty myself." In describing symptoms and their readings here, I am imposing a kind of stylistic formality on what is often a very fluid and changeable system of reading body signs as a part of enacting bodies.

Samoans experience symptoms from a pool of body signs. This symptom pool describes the range of signs the body makes, but no body signal is by definition negative or positive, good or bad. Rather, the principles of this symptom pool establish the criteria for treating a sign as either a symptom of illness or of health. There are four basic categories of signs which make up this pool of readable body properties: signs of the movement of substances or their obstruction, body mobility or its impairment, emotional propriety or deviance, and the condition of the skin. Both MacPherson and MacPherson [1990:158-189], and Forsyth [1983:123-141 *passim*] distinguish body signs by where in the body the symptom is located, because in each case they were focussing on what is physically done to the body in the healing process. My discussion here focusses on the principles of proper body function, which are implicated in symptoms, and so, differs from, and adds a new dimension to, these previous descriptions.

The healthy body is a body through which substances flow freely. Blood, urine, sweat, menses, and phlegm are scrutinized as signs of either good health, or impending illness. Bowels should be free, urine should be expelled in considerable quantity and with great force, phlegm should be easily coughed out and should be of the consistency of normal saliva or semen, and blood, either in menstruation or from injury, should flow easily, and be consistently bright red in colour.

Mobility of limbs, and of the torso, is also important in Samoan health, the healthy body being fluid in movement, with no pain associated even with strenuous exertion. Limbs and the spine are observed for their flexibility, and painlessness of movement, and for changes in the shape and orientation of the limb when at rest.

The meanings of emotional or behaviourial signs derive, in part, from the concern Samoans have with propriety and humility. Expressions of extreme emotions, even in situations of extraordinary stress, are avoided. The healthy person is a calm one. Intense emotional outbursts are punishable, if not associated with illness.[8] From the age of 3 or 4 onward, children learn to be restrained in their emotional expressions, and to be cautious in admitting to heightened emotional distress [Ochs 1988:145-168; Gerber 1875:157-163].

The final core focus in this physical vocabulary is the boundary of the body with the world, the skin. Healthy skin is skin which sweats freely, and is clear of blemishes and staining scars, other than those voluntarily imbedded such as tattoos. It is warm to the touch in infants, and cool in children and adults, with a clear even colour. Skin is permeable, and substances can pass both into, and out of the body through the skin. Any indication of impairment of this aspect of healthy skin is understood as a symptom of illness. Indeed, so important are skin signs, they are the most elaborately developed category of symptom in Samoan diagnosis. While MacPherson and MacPherson [1990:163] suggest the skin's importance is a function of its vulnerability, because of exposure to injury or the elements, many of my informants commented that skin is important because, in one man's words, "everything a person is doing is on his skin for me to see." Skin, for Samoans is the ultimate and most intimate point of connection with the world, and at its most crucial, it is the only reliable "text" for other Samoans to read the nature and quality of some other person. Skin is the public organ, beneath which inscrutable private processes occur, and so attention to the skin serves as an act of surveillance over the inner workings of the body itself.

Within this pool of symptom classes, body signs are interpreted based on what they tell the observer about the functioning of the body. Emanating from these classes of symptom types, Samoans can construct elaborate clusters of body signs. It begins with such higher order signs as laboured breathing and the absence of phlegm; fever and discoloration of the skin; impaired bowel movements or painful urination; skin eruptions or discolorations not accompanied by fever; pain in limbs, either of the bone or muscle or joint, all of which are the same kind of pain conceptually; or pain in the head or in internal organs such as heart or liver pain.

Unlike Western medicine, the range of symptoms is relatively simple. They are classified in terms of the four conceptual foundations of body signs—movement and flow, appropriate expression, spatial orientation, and the condition of the skin as a link between the body and the world, since Samoans are remarkably economical in their explanations and rationalizations of events in the world. As well, the absence of a specialist healer class in Samoa, and the Samoan concept of expertise as being about success in practice rather than about information or specialized knowledge, has meant that healers are not in a position to develop elaborate models as an exercise in specialization or secrecy. Since medical knowledge is also common knowledge, there has been no legitimate intellectual space available for the development of an elaborate and specialized system of medical explanation [see also MacPherson and MacPherson 1990:101].

But within this limited range of higher order symptoms, there are what might be called the children of the body sign, elaborate clusters of symptoms defined by such things as order of emergence, intensity, and changes in where the signs of body function and distress are manifesting themselves. There is also substantial richness in Samoan understandings of the connections between body function and symptoms. For example, fever has many causes and effects, reflected in the several different explanations of fever in different illness cases:

- movement of internal organs blocks the flow of fluid in the body, trapping it in the skin where it overheats.
- fluid becomes overheated by becoming blocked around an organ, the heat then passing through to the skin.
- organs themselves become overheated when effected by disease, and pass this heat through to the skin.
- fluids themselves have a property of heat which becomes agitated during overexertion, during illness and because of some malfeasance or minor crime
- fluids in the skin pass heat from outside the body to the organs which take on the heat. A diseased organ or an organ not in its proper place cannot take up this heat which then remains in the fluid passing by the skin.
- the body has a limited capacity to cool itself. Inappropriate behaviour, from being immodest to simply staying in the sun too long, can overwhelm this capacity. For example, many people told me that blushing is a kind of localized fever associated with immodesty or minor misbehaviour.
- finally, but not exhaustively, connected to this is the relationship between fever and cure. Fever was often described as a positive and necessary process whereby the excess heat from the

organs effected by disease was passed out of the body, where urination and sweating are either inadequate or impaired.

While the pool of available symptoms is simple and quite general in character, the range of both the causes and of the things symptoms explain or at least indicate is quite extensive, and more often than not vigorously disputed, by people involved with an ill person.

Higher order "parent" symptoms, simple in general outline, are complicated by their collation into what I referred to above as "child symptom sets," an image which was suggested to me by a Samoan healer, who, in describing a person's illness and death while under treatment at the national hospital, commented that, "the doctors didn't understand that the pain in his head, that was the father of his death, but it was the children, his heart and his bowels, that killed him. They only saw the father, and forgot to think about the children." These sets are clusters of symptoms defined by their associations with each other, their intensity, and their order of appearance in the patient. Determining the history of these symptom clusters is a means of determining, at least initiually, the source of the illness, and of predicting, again in a preliminary way, the path the illness will likely take. For example, a combination of fever, headache and vomiting can, in different order, be evidence of different diseases. A fever followed rapidly by a blinding headache and then vomiting, is a disease of the head, in which over exposure to the sun is the most probable cause. Vomiting, fever, and the slow onset of a steady, but low grade headache on the other hand is evidence of heart failure, or the collapse of the *manava*. Death is likely, as breathing finally collapses from the combination of insufficient food, and the inability of the body to cool itself properly. Finally, a headache of sudden onset, followed by vomiting and fever, is a cluster associated with thinking bad thoughts about ancestors. This ordering of the onset of signs tells the patient and those around her much about the nature of the illness, the play of organs and processes, both biological and social, and the likely paths to recovery.

All diseases are considered in terms of the cluster of symptoms which appear, and each symptom is evidence of a particular obstruction or malfunction. The disease is defined by these combinations, and not the individual attributes of symptoms alone. However, this also sounds more formal and fixed than it is in practice. It is better to think of child symptom sets as an available catalogue of possibilities, rather than a formal and fixed classification of illness signs. So much of the evidence of these sets of symptoms, from their severity, to the order of their onset, is open to either direct manipulation or to misinterpretation, that it would be inaccurate to think of this as a single, formal, catalogue of illness attributes. The interpretation of these symptoms is never inexorable or pre-ordained

[MacPherson and MacPherson 1990:193]. Symptoms are signals, whether signifiers as in skin eruptions, effects following from impairment of organs, such as breathing difficulties or headaches, or the manifestation of organ obstruction or organ movement, as in visceral pain, constipation, or the inability to ejaculate. Within the framework of the conceptual pool of body signs I described above, illness signs can be read, misread or ignored, making the classification and fixed definition of symptoms analytically difficult, if not impossible. Table 1 gives some examples of illnesses by general class and symptom cluster, but with this warning in mind—symptoms can be completely ignored during diagnosis, either by deception on the part of the patient, or by misdirection on the part of the *fofō*.

Illness in Samoa is, in most people's perceptions, endemic, and is a constant concern. Government statistics list the most common cause of death as pneumonic influenza [about 60% of all reported deaths in 1985 — Samoa Department of Statistics 1990 Annual Report]. Although Baker and Crews do not analyze cause of death data from Samoa, because of its unreliability, they compare Samoa with American Samoa, and suggest the leading pathological cause of death in the Samoas is cardiovascular disease [1986:98*ff*]. However, my informants felt that the leading cause of death was simply old age. "The person wears out, has no more strength left and so she dies," I was told. The average age at death for reported deaths in 1989 was 72 years for women and 69 for men [per.comm. Samoan Department of Health]. For my informants the most dangerous illnesses for adults, both male and female, are, in order of concern, diabetes [*ma'i suka*], *aitu* attack [*ma'i aitu*], cancer [*kanesa*], and a generic category labelled *ma'i fatu* or heart disease. Many of my informants also expressed concern over hypertension [*toto maualuga*, literally high or proud blood]. The do not consider it a disease, but see it, instead, as a side effect of arrogance. In children the most common illness and cause of death informants reported was asthma, for which they use the English word at all times, and which encompassed almost every manifestation of bronchial distress in children. Similar symptoms in adults are diagnosed as either heart disease or cancer. Infant death is most often attributed to *aitu* attack, the second leading concern being malformed lungs and heart. Samoans are vigilant, carefully watching for signs of these illnesses in themselves, and in the people around them.

Another class of symptom distinctions, those related to mental disorders, is not extremely well developed in Samoan illness models [Clement 1974]. There are two types of mental disorder. The first, *valea*, refers to emotional and behaviourial deviations, including insanity and derangement. The term *valea* is also applied to derangements of intellectual function, such as conditions comparable to dissociative disorders, and to normative states of derangement, such as grief. A phrase, *ma'i valea* [and according

Class of Illness	Parent Symptom	Examples, with symptom progression
Heart and Blood	Ma'i fatu - impairment of blood and breath flow through the lungs, heart and stomach	Uaumini [varicose veins] - pain in legs, swelling, emergence of discoloured veins Ma'i oso [stroke] - confusion followed closely by headache and then collapse, paralysis and "stupid muscles
Skin	Lafa tane - marks on the skin	Ma'sua [sick sore] - pain then reddening of a point in the skin, emergence of a boil, explosive expulsion of pus latolo [sores on infant's head] - crying, tossing of head, development of non-pustulant sores, scabbbing and a spread of sores
Viscera	Manava - impairment of steady flow of food, substances through gut	Papala [ulcer] - loss of appetite, cramping, crippling pain, bloody vomit, discoloration of eyes, dark urine

Table 1: Some Samoan illness sites, higher order symptom classes, and their associated symptom clusters.

to some informants *ma'i valea o le aitu,* emotion illness caused by ghosts or spirits] is sometimes applied to longstanding mental derangements. A woman who lived in and around the streets of Apia, unwashed and obsessively cleaning litter and rubble from the streets and roadways, was often described to me as having a "*valea* [mental derangement] sickness," but the generality of the term's application suggests that mental disorder is not formally codified. Forsyth [1983:135*ff*] has described in great detail Samoan practices surrounding mental disorder, and her conclusions on the formal classification of derangement parallel mine, to the effect that mental disorder is not readily distinguished from other forms of simple behaviourial deviance such as

> displaying "crazy," "stupid" behaviour; offending your parents [which] can cause one to feel sad [depression]; failure to respect one's elders [e.g., the *matai*] can cause one to feel guilty [hostility, aggression, anger]; and behaving anti-socially because one has a "sore heart" [anger, hurt, antisocial, manic, depress(ed)] [Forsyth date:135].

The other classification of mental derangement is *mea ua lēatoa ai le tino* [literally the unwholeness or incompleteness of the body], and is applied to retardation and to physical deformities or handicaps, which appear to always have a component of mental disability attached to them. That is, a person with some form of cerebral palsy, is, by definition rather than by diagnosis, deemed to be mentally disabled as well. These disorders are understood to be the result of malformation of the brain and its linkages to the *manava* [heart-lung-stomach] structure which, in fully formed bodies provides the physical material of the brain, and regenerates it on a regular basis. These deformities are usually caused by *aitu* attack. The mentally retarded are treated with deference and even considered to by some to be specially blessed. A school for handicapped children, the *Fia Malamalama* [making light/knowledge] School, was opened in the late 1980's, to accomodate the care and education of moderately retarded and physically handicapped children. While it had about 17 or 18 regular students during my time in Samoa, there was a general sense among Samoans I spoke with that the school was a nice thing to do, but not necessary since families care well for those members too infirm to care for themselves. As one woman explained "maybe they want to make them work like everyone else, but the person with handicaps cannot do that, and others should care for them and not force them to feed pigs or dig taro or weave mats." While the handicapped are not absolved from adhering to rules of proper behaviour, they are not criticized for their inability to perform regular daily work, nor are they blamed for their condition. However, people with *valea* disorders are often subjected to intense criticism, and even punishment, if the cause of their disorder is not determined to be from random *aitu* attack or some socially acceptable form of temporary derangement, such as grief.

There is another form of psychological distress which is not considered an illness, but a normal, though dangerous, organic condition[9]: *musu*. There is no English equivalent for this word, or the state it names. Informants would translate the word as either sadness or anger, an indication of the complexity of these concepts rather than the ambiguity of *musu*. *Musu* is a special form of emotion, where the person becomes withdrawn and quiet, tends to avoid all human contact, and often withdraws some distance from the living core of the village, occasionally spending time alone in the bush. MacPherson and MacPherson [1990:194-195] and Freeman [1983:218-219] describe *musu* as a form of frustration safety valve, since sufferers have often recently experienced some disappointment, or other thwarted expectation. *Musu* allows Samoans a socially positive space to withdraw into in order to reorient their emotions and expectations, consistent with the negative attitude toward acts done in private as anti-social under other circumstances. However, my own direct experience, which is admittedly limited to fewer than two dozen instances suggest this may be the case in some, but by no means all instances of *musu*. *Musu* appears to be an expression of quite a wide range of psycho-traumatic experiences and conditions, type 1 manic-depression, and rapid cycling type 2 manic depression.[10]

While the person in *musu* is considered temporarily deranged, he or she is not considered sick. No effort is made to interfere, unless the state lasts longer than one or two days, and the person is not queried about the cause of the event when it is over. However, people in *musu* are at special risk for illness or *aitu* attack, because their attention is impaired, and so, villagers and family members will, surreptitiously, keep close surveillance on someone in *musu*. I found *musu* troubling, and even frightening, because it can occur very suddenly, in one case between one sentence and another in a conversation with a young man who had been telling me about his mother's work for the local Catholic church. *Musu* may allow a space for frustration to be redirected, and so serve as an internal or personal release, but it also acts as a break on the behaviour of others, a signal that impositions of obligation or authority may have become excessive. Because it puts the person in this state in danger of illness, people are aware that they should not put a person into a state of *musu* by their own actions, such as greed, rudeness or anger, and that their demands on others should be reasonable and fair. This reinforces the practices of deference, respect, sharing, and humility in which individual bodies are implicated in complex and perilous ways. That is to say, the *musu* of a teenaged girl can chastise even the most powerful of *matai*.

Physically, there are four general sites of illnesses in, or on the body. Illness can be sited in the emotions. Emotions reside in the gut and are felt in the gut as disturbances or pains. Illness be located in the limbs, or the peripheral organs such as the kidneys, pain in which is often understood as evidence of anger at someone, for example. Illness can occur in or on the skin, that is, at the surface which encompasses the body as a whole, and through which connections with the world are expressed and recorded. Finally, illness can happen in the core of the body, in the *manava* [heart-lung], the *to'ala*, the stomach, and in the brain or genitals.

Along with these discrete sites, illness can have one of five causal models. Overexertion or overexposure to sun or heat is the most common organic explanation for illness. More often than not illness which result from this kind of excess are considered artifacts of carelessness, and carry little or no blame. Misbehaviour, including, but not restricted to crimes, anger, disobedience or lack of respect, and failure to show proper reverence to ancestors, are the second most common cause of illnesses among Samoans. The social controlling function of this category of illnesses is obvious, but at the same time, blame and obligation with respect to behaviour related illness is rebuttable. Literally, in the process of diagnosis during which a malfeasance is suspected of being the cause, the patient or her family can enter and defend a plea of not guilty. *Aitu* illness, that is illness or impairment caused by *aitu* attack, can be divided into two forms. One results from socially inappropriate behaviour of a more abstract sort such as immodesty or excessive pride, and the other from the capricious malice or anger of the *aitu* themselves.[11] Schoeffel [1978:412-414] notes that *aitu* illness is more common among women, something explained by my informants by the physical vulnerability of the internal organs, which are more readily accessible in women, through the vagina. However I could find no consensus on the issue of why women are more prone to *aitu* attack than men. Part of this lack of consensus may be related to the somewhat ambiguous ranking of genders, with women accruing greater generic status than men based on their gendered position. As such, it may be that Samoans are more concerned with, even fearful, of women's illnesses because the stakes are higher when a woman becomes ill given their role in the central identificatory concern with the reproduction of family, and family ties. A further complication to *aitu* illness is that these spirit beings are also known to work as agents for ancestors, for example, an extra-corporeal *soa* relationship in which the *aitu* themselves have no motive, but are expressing and carrying out the objective of some other entity. Samoans also have a limited micro-organism causative model. These organisms exist in such places as the dew laden cloud forests which surmount the central mountain ridges of the islands and enter the body accidentally, usually causing problems in fluid flow or, if there are sufficient numbers, forcing organs from their normal positions. These organisms or substances have no sentience, though a persons behaviour can put them at greater risk of "infection." Finally, there are the *ma'i palagi* or European diseases, such as cancer, diabetes or flu, which have, conceptually at least, a senseless and de-socialized causation occuring somewhat randomly. I say somewhat, because a predisposition to *palagi* illness is often read as evidence of some social problem, which is at the heart of the illness event. That is, although *ma'i palagi* are, as a class of illnesses, blameless there is likely to be a trigger in the patients or her families behaviour or history which has rendered them vulnerable to these diseases. Whatever the ultimate organic causes of illness, there is always some element of social disrepute or disrepair in the illness process which governs the shape of this process as it is played out in the body of the patient and in the body of the social world to which he or she is attached.

Illnesses have paths through which the state of the body passes on its way from illness to health again. Depending on the child symptom cluster at the heart of the illness, these paths can take several forms. The most common is an intensification of symptoms, followed by the addition of new symptoms, followed finally by the return to a reading of body signs as normal. In Samoan illness paths, symptoms do not disappear so much as they change. Through the course of the cure, Samoans expect not only an intensification of the symptoms they have presented with, but also expect new symptoms to emerge as signs they are healing. This expectation of additional symptoms as signs of healing is reflected in the sale of over the counter analgesics in Samoa. While tablet forms of most common analgesic compounds are available throughout the islands, most Samoans prefer analgesics in powdered bicarbonate of soda. I found this curious, because most people who I asked about their drug choices told me they disliked the taste of such products as Disprin, an ASA-based bicarbonate compound imported from Australia. However, they went on to explain that they could tell the Disprin was working because it made them belch. The sign of the success of the drug was not the elimination of the headache, which came with time as well, but the other symptoms the medication effected on the body.

The basic path of all illnesses is a return to normal activity and to normal body signs, even though in some instances these signs are impossible to distinguish from illness symptoms on casual observation. Phlegm is one such symptom. While normal phlegm production is considered a sign of health, where normal is understood as easily expelled and meeting certain criteria regarding colour and texture, illness related phlegm is defined mostly in terms of its relationship to some other symptom. It is not uncommon for someone to comment on a phlegmatic cough as a sign the person is very ill, and then to comment some days later on a cough which has, to all intents, not changed, as signalling the person is once again healthy. What has intervened in those several days is a path of healing in which the meaning of signs from the body, and the experience of that signalling body, have been transformed, by the person's progress along a route of cure.

The body, then, is closely attended to within a framework of understandings about how the body works. Illness is not simply an organic event to which a model of the body is applied so much as it is part of living that model. Illnesses and symptom classes, while generally understood and generally shared, are experiential rather than a priori. Within this framework of possibilities, the processes of diagnosis and curing are carried out.

Seeing the Illness:
Diagnosis and Agreement

Understanding diagnostic practice is a cornerstone of much of the work in medical anthropology. In the arts and disciplines of diagnosis, the web of embodiment is at is most crucial and, perhaps, most explicitly complex, because in the process of diagnosis, the entire range of practices through which the body is constituted are enacted in a space of emergency and concern. The imperiled body is not simply an object deformed by disease or injury. As Lewis [1977] has noted, the ill body in many societies is a mimetic dialogue between the organic wellbeing of the person and the social wellbeing of the community. In many societies bodies alone do not get sick: persons, communities, and relationships are implicated in the illness that afflicts the organic body. This is the case in Samoa. Illness is always about a concern for the wellbeing of the community as a whole. "Ken can never be well again," a woman told me after a young cousin was taken to the National Hospital after collapsing while climbing a coconut tree. "His family has a sickness from all their anger, and they need to take this medicine instead if Ken is going to stop being sick." Although their models of illness aetiology allow for random, unmotivated disease, it is in the process of diagnosis that this determination is made. What is always at stake in diagnosis is not simply the body of the patient, but the body of relations and obligations, which may be diseased as well. The clinical encounter in Samoa is not only about Ken's pneumonia, but about the preservation of society by the protection and preservation of relationships among persons. The clinical encounter in Samoa is an act of profound importance in enculturing the world.

Formal diagnosis is actually the third step in the path illnesses take, illustrated in Figure 8.1. Illnesses are first recognized by the potential patient, in their attention to their own body signs. Recall that body signs need not be disease symptoms, so this attention to the talkative body involves a calculated rehearsal of recent and even distantly removed behaviour in order to give the sign context, and possibly transform it into a symptom. Because illness will more than likely impugn the quality or nature of a person's social behaviour, there is a resistance to reading signs as signals of illness, and even obvious symptoms are often initially ignored, both by the patient and those around her. This attention to bodily signals for evidence of illness is an ongoing, persistent and complex process involving both the individual and the people around them. The second phase, which marks the public start of an illness event, comes with the observation of symptoms by others. Efforts to avoid the observation of symptoms by others cannot be overstressed. Illness can directly, and negatively, affect a family, in their relations in the wider *'āiga*, or village. It is during this phase that self care is often initiated, either with herbal concoctions, or over the counter drugs. There is an advantage in keeping the illness secret, and treating it in silence and privacy. The presence of an alternative, non-blaming healing tradition, the Western hospital and clinic based system, allows for greater secrecy and deception than was, perhaps, possible in the past. Indeed, because many over the counter medications effectively mask symptoms, it is possible to be very sick, and have no one observe this fact. The regular, and extensive use of over the counter analgesics, antihistamines, decongestants, antipyretics, and antitussives, because they can disguise symptoms, are examples of the masking possibilities which Western medicine has afforded. One man put it quite explicitly when he came to borrow some pain tablets from me. I asked him what was wrong, and he told me he was sick, but wanted no one to know until he had a chance to return the rugby shoes he had stolen from another man's house. Denying illness is an important aspect of the illness process in Samoa. Through denial, or other efforts to hide symptoms, the ill person is seeking to preserve her social integrity and dignity, an integrity and dignity which is expressed in, with, and because of the socially configured body the patient is enacting.

An illness which does not respond to this treatment, or which is obviously serious enough to warrant more skilful intervention, is classified as to its cultural origins, as either *ma'i Samoa* or *ma'i palagi* [European disease], and the patient is either brought to the National Hospital, or local clinic, for Western care, or a *fofō* is called in to examine the patient's illness and social behaviours. Today the presence and accessibility of Western care is less important for its control of infectious disease, as it is, in the eyes of my informants, for providing an avenue of diagnosis and care which avoids the social perils of having a sick person call into question the propriety of a family's social relations. Many of my informants were quite explicit in explaining that, initially, they prefer to treat almost any disease as amenable to *palagi* care, to avoid calling in a *fofō*, whose presence and diagnosis risks family honour and status. This practice of reframing illness includes reclassifying some illnesses formally included in the *ma'i Samoa* category as *ma'i palagi*, the most common being to simply call whatever illness one may have the "flu." Influenza is the most reported cause of death by family members, followed by old age, both of which are considered blameless illnesses and deaths. Death statistics, and indeed epidemiological data on disease prevalence in Samoa is often difficult to decipher and more often than not is unreliable, at least epidemiologically, because so many other factors are involved in accepting and announcing a particular diseases presence.

Formal diagnosis by *fofō*, the third phase in the illness path, takes many forms. The first step in all diagnosis involves a close scrutiny of the patient's body, to determine what the outward signs of the disease may be. This may be as simple as examining all parts of the body's surface for illness signs, such as skin eruptions, blisters, or swellings. It may involve an examination of body fluids, including small amounts of blood drawn from the foot or hand, and close examination of faeces, urine, saliva, or menstrual blood. Limbs are often manipulated to examine their flexibility, and range of motion, and orifices may be superficially probed for obstructions or malformations. A more formal kind of physical examination, the exploratory massage, may be undertaken to map the location and size of the internal organs. This massage can be very detailed, and take several hours to complete. At the end of all this, the *fofō* has a complete picture of the state of the body and its parts.

Throughout this physical examination the healer maintains a running interrogation of the patient, and family members, who offer their own observations on the patient's condition and behaviour leading up to the onset of the illness, and during its initial progress. The clinical encounter is public event, one in which entire families, and even large segments of villages, may take part. It is carried out in the home of the sick person rather than at some special healing location, although in the case of minor ailments, patients may travel with family members to the home of the *fofō*, out of courtesy to the age of most successful healers.

This physical examination, and organic clinical history, is the first step in what, in most cases, is a two part process of diagnosis. Unless the illness can be immediately determined to be organic in nature, such as those caused by Samoan micro-organisms, injury, or overexertion, the healer concludes the clinical investigation with a detailed cross examination of the patient, and his or her family. The *fofō* inquires about the patient's relations with those around theme, about their behaviour toward others, both living and dead, and about any misdemeanours, or more serious offenses, any member of the family may have committed. What is observed and interpreted in the clinical encounter is not simply the actual manifestations of illness on the body, but the connections between these manifestations, and social problems in which the patient is actually involved or at least implicated by relationships with others. From this intensive clinical examination, the healer makes a preliminary determination of the nature of the disease, and its likely cause, and begins the plan of therapy the

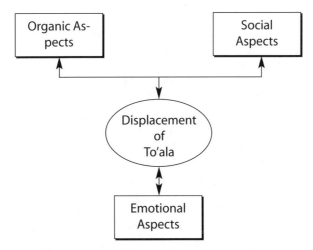

Figure 8.3 Some clinical determinations in the diagnosis of a disorder of the to'ala.

patient and family will need to follow. Figure 8.3 illustrates the range of findings a healer may make with respect to a disorder of the *to'ala*, the stomach-heart of Samoan anatomy. The *fofō* looks for organic manifestations of organ displacement or strangulation of some other other, since the *to'ala* is notorious for moving or being moved, and effecting by pressure or ligature the functioning of other organs. At the same time, the healer discerns problems within or between families or individuals, disobedience or even more serious social breaches such as crime. Finally, the *fofō* is looking for emotional and even cognitive disruptions in the individual, picking out such things as a break down in the persons sense of trust or security, fears and anxieties, and perhaps the most important emotional component, guilt.

What the healer looks for is disorder, not only within the body, but in the social world around the patient. The healer is looking for things out of place which are no longer following the appropriate paths of humility, deference, and communal responsibility. The healer looks for this, not only in the relations of flow and movement within the body, but also in the relations of obligation and compliance around the imperiled person. The other participants in this examination engage in a process of negotiation, and sometimes open contestation, of the direction both of the questions asked, and the diagnosis which is arrived at. Family members will deny or contest assertions of malfeasance on the part of either the patient or other family members, will offer different diagnostic suggestions in response to the *fofō's* clinical observations and, in extreme cases, will actually deny the accuracy of the diagnosis, and seek another healer for consultation. In the Samoan clinical encounter, a complex process of arbitration and interpretation is engaged. The expert cannot impose determinations. The information adduced in the examination is subject to different analyses and readings, and the process of the specific disease is literally invented, and reinvented, in an effort to arrive at a successful diagnosis, that is, a diagnosis with the greatest likelihood of effective cure, with the least damage to the patient and the relations around them.

Anatomy, symptoms, etiological hypotheses, and surveillance conjoin in the clinical encounter. The observers, both healer and the patient's relations, are looking for changes and extraordinary signs. They are looking for extreme expressions of normal body functions, body motion, and of behaviour. Restraint and not "showing off," are at the core of Samoan humility, and in a very real sense, the clinical encounter is looking for a lack of humility in the body, that is, a body which is exaggerated in its expressions and substances. The healer is also looking for a lack of strength, because a body that cannot endure the normal rigour of daily life is a dangerous body. It can no longer be depended upon to meet its obligations, and comport itself with modesty and propriety. Healing, which continues the process of clinical investigation while restoring the body to its humble, dignified, stillness, addresses, in the enactment of the patient's progression back to health, a re-incorporation of these core precepts of dignity, humility, and strength.

The process of diagnosis is the riskiest moment in Samoan embodiment. In Figure 8.1 I have represented a fluctuation in the level of dignity attached to the body in the illness event. At the point of formal diagnosis, the body is at its lowest ebb of social dignity, because it, and the people around it, are at the greatest risk. The objective of this entire process is to begin to return the body to an appropriate state of dignity and status, in itself, and in its relation vis à vis others.

Treatment and Restoration: Making the Body Whole in the Body of Society

Once a diagnosis and cause is agreed upon, the patient and the family begin the process of treatment determined by the *fofō*. Because aetiologies vary, there are several paths this treatment may take, although the objective, the restoration of orderliness and propriety, is the same.

Aitu illnesses, whether organic disorders, displaced organs, or full blown *aitu* possession, require the most detailed form of healing, because not only must the physical condition of the body be addressed, the offended *aitu* or the ancestor or other spirit, including Saints, Jesus, or the Christian God, must be appeased [Goodman 1971; Mageo 1991]. While there are some formulaic recitations a healer may use in dealing with particular *aitu*, these are quite rare, usually only applied to the more vicious and powerful *aitu* known as *teine*, or to specific kinds of ailments in which *aitu* are always implicated [Moyle 1974:163-177]. Most often the treatment of *aitu*-caused illnesses involves apologizing to the offended spirit and promising not to commit the offense again in the future. The apology may be verbal, and may be either public or private, depending on the severity of the illness, and the danger the *aitu* poses to others. It may also take the form of clearing away weeds from a site where *aitu* are known to live or travel, or cleaning the grave site of an ancestor who has been offended by lack of attention. In extreme cases, regular obeisances, such as prayers, may be ordered for both the patient and their family, along with restrictions on going to certain places or engaging in certain activities, such as courting or gardening in particular plantations, or sections of bush.

Along with these obeisances and apologies for *aitu* illness, Samoan curing of all types of illness includes two other forms of organic treatment: massage [*fofō*] and herbal cures combined with psychological counselling [*taulāsea*]. Forsyth [1983:151-154] describes these two types of treatments as specialists, but both my advisors, and MacPherson and MacPherson [1990:116-120], insist that the terms refer to types of healing practices, and not to distinctions between practitioners themselves. The term *fofō* is also used as the generic term for traditional healers in everyday conversation, the more formal and proper term *taulāsea* used in formal conversations. No one I spoke with distinguished healers by type of treatment used. Rather, healers were distinguished by the illnesses they were best at treating. While some *fofō* use either massage or herbal/counselling techniques exclusively, this is a function of the illnesses they are best at treating, and not of specialist classes of treatment experts. All *fofō* are versed in both methods, as are most adult Samoans. While both men and women are *fofō*, women appear to be in the majority. This is likely a function of the connection Samoans make between women and the maintenance, and most especially, the preservation and restoration of social orderliness and propriety.

Massage has as its objective the restoration of organs to their proper location, and the opening of pathways for substances and energy to flow freely through the body. Massage is intensive and often quite painful, a form of visceral chiropractic, in which organs are moved often considerable distances within the gut. The art of massage in Samoa is very well developed. An experienced healer can massage the uterus or womb in such a way as to prevent pregnancy, returning it to its normal position when the couple determines to have another child. Samoan massage experts have considerable skill in setting broken bones, in freeing up fluid accumulated in the lungs, and in helping patients to pass gall and kidney stones.

Samoan massage, as MacPherson and MacPherson [1990] and Forsyth [1983] note, is recognized by Western trained medical personnel as being remarkable for both the range of conditions it treats, and for its effectiveness. I was told by two doctors visiting from New Zealand that it is not uncommon for *fofō* experienced in bone setting massage [*fogau*] to be flown to New Zealand and Australia to help train doctors and therapists in these techniques. While in Samoa, I fractured a bone in my wrist. I was treated with massage while the injury healed. On my return to Canada, I had my wrist examined by my personal physician, who remarked on both the seriousness of the fracture, and the skill with which it had been set and treated.

The other form of treatment involves a combination of herbal concoctions, the application of leaves or other plants to body parts, and psychological counselling or "talking cures" [Kinloch 1985; MacPherson and MacPherson 1990:202-203]. The herbal treatments, almost all of which are derived from common plants which require no special skill at harvesting, are for the most part emetics and purgatives of varying degrees of strength [Cox and Banack 1991:147-168]. The healer may bring these ingredients to the diagnosis, and begin preparing them while detailing any other steps the cure must take. They may also simply leave the family with instructions for where to gather the plants, what proportions and what methods to use to prepare the medicine, and how to administer it. Gathering is usually left to older children, while preparation and administration is carried out by the patient's mother or other close female relative, except for treatments of the male genitals, which are self administered. The progress of the treatment changes as the disease changes, and instructions will be left for what changes to make in the medication during the course of the illness. In most cases, the healer does not follow the progression of the cure, unless called upon by the family during the course of the treatment because of problems, the manifestation of symptoms not expected or, in some cases, for public reassurance that the cure is proceeding properly.

At the same time that the healer prepares his or her medication, or prepares the instructions, he or she begins the process of the "talking cure" as well. This is most often a kind of lecture on proper behaviour, peppered with questions to the patient, or the patient's family, about what proper behaviour and proper values are. The patient and their family are enjoined to apologize for even the smallest misdemeanour, and to recognize the importance of social responsibilities, even in cases which have a simple organic cause. As one healer explained, "even *palagi* sickness is sometimes a punishment or an attack because the person has been bad." After the initial diagnostic encounter, the talking cure is carried on by the family, who are enjoined by the healer, to remind the patient of their responsibilities and the basic values of *Fa'a Samoa*. In some instances the patient and the family may be required to seek additional counselling from their Christian minister, or to take time during the *sā* [the evening prayer] to discuss this illness, and to remind themselves of the proper way to avoid such events in the future.

The ultimate path a treatment will take depends on the linkages between symptoms and causes, and the progress of healing is closely monitored by the family for the effectiveness of the cure. Quiet, stillness, and a cool space to rest are strictly enforced, and all villagers will endeavour to restrain their activities around the house of a sick person, thus directly participating in the curing process. This participation is not only kindness, but an expression of the interest all community members have in the success of the cure. "When Ioane was ill during the independence holiday, we were all worried because we wondered why God was angry at [our village]" one man told me. "He had hurt the little girl which was his bad thing, but he had done it here, and so it was our bad thing too."

Dignity and order are finally restored when the patient emerges in daily life as a normal and full participant in his or her obligations. The long process of the cure, its slow progression through new symptoms, are all signs of a return of dignity and harmony. The family, and even the entire village, return to a state of propriety, with the return of the patient as a healthy functioning body deployed with modesty, decorum and strength. The patient is not isolated, and there is no secrecy surrounding the illness and its progress, once it has been publicly recognized. There is no special kingdom of the sick in Samoa [cf Sontag 1978].

Illness in Samoa is about protecting, preserving, and restoring good and proper bodies, individually and in their social relationships, through surveillance and discipline. In Samoa, illness is also talk. The most common topic of conversation, even with almost total strangers, is the state of one's health, or the health of the people you know. Illness talk, wide ranging and unrestricted, maintains the body by the discipline of its questions and comments. Illness talk makes the healthy body a disciplined, surveilled body, as readily and actively as banishment or toilet training or learning the appropriate meanings of food.

Illness, Healing and the Work of Proper Bodies

Health and illness in Samoa are practices of vigilance and discipline. They entail on all bodies a rigorous, though never rigid, set of obligations and expectations about how and why the body works the way it does, and how these aspects of the body's functioning connect with obligations and responsibilities at the heart of social life. Health is a strategy, a form of deployment, and a process of attention, in which the body enacted is also the body queried and examined. As such, health is a form of fundamental awareness in which the practices of embodiment are implicated at the very core of participation in the world.

Health and illness in Samoa are part of a larger, and always evolving concern for the fundamental precepts of dignity and humility and strength. Illness diminishes dignity, renders the body special and immodest, and saps endurance, depleting the body's ability to move with good and proper authority and honour. Illness also diminishes social order and cohesiveness, because the risk in illness is never simply the risk to the patient herself. It is not so much that in Samoa disease occurs at the level of the community, though in practical terms that is certainly so. Rather, disease in Samoa is always about the implications for order, propriety, and civility which follow from the disabling of any individual member. So all encompassing is this embodied concern for social connection that the incapacitation of any part needs to be accounted for in the network of disqualifications extending outward into the patients world of social engagement. Illness practice intensifies this commitment to propriety and communal connection by putting the entire system at risk. While Western models of disease have deflected blame inward onto the individual, Samoan disease practice deploys the individual body as a special kind of statute which empowers civility and communal interest in the pain and recovery of each individual member. It also reinforces the centrality of communal interest in the embodied experience of the individual, who must rely on the restoration of social order for his or her own, individual, return to health and well-being.

In linking the practice of healthy bodies to the wider concerns of appropriate space, and the proper deployment of reverent still bodies in the social field, illness enables and authorizes each member of the Samoan community to directly effect the proper course of society, and to sustain and strengthen the social whole through the process of strengthening the body, endangered by illness and injury. Illness suffuses the social world with risk, and in doing so, empowers the individual as the fundamental and indivisible particle because of which this social world persists and prospers.

Pita recovered very slowly, following intervention by three *fofō*, each with special skills in different aspects of the *aitu* attack which had debilitated his body, and threatened his life. Over the days which followed his attack, members of his *'āiga* spent long hours examining their relationships with his mother and his brother, offering apologies and gifts as signs of concern and consideration. A cousin who had delighted in accusing Pita of being a *fa'afafine,* because, he said, Pita's muscles were too soft and weak, presented him with a new pair of rugby shoes, which cost him almost three month's wages. The Methodist minister exhorted the families of Pita's *'āiga* to show special care in all their relations. Pita's mother and brother visited relatives, bringing small gifts, and making apologies for any slight they might have inflicted. Eventually, Pita emerged from his house, thinner, and physically weaker, but, socially, he was stronger than he had ever been in his life.

Chapter 9

Changes in Directions/The Directions of Change in Making Proper Samoan Bodies

This book has often travelled along a landscape of abstraction, even though throughout what I have been talking about are real bodies, in a real place and time, doing real things in order to invent and move in and around a real world. I have done this because my objective here is more theoretical than it is empirical, if such an analytic division can sustained. As I said at the outset, this book is not Samoa, it is an anthropology of the body in Samoa. Without repudiating that intention, this chapter looks at several instances of sociopolitical and cultural transformation underway in Samoa today in order to show how an approach to Samoan culture, and by extension to any culture anywhere, grounded in an understanding of local processes of embodiment, can help understand and perhaps even explain larger scale historical transformations. What I want to address here are changes, and some subtle shifts in direction, which are effecting and being effected by embodied praxis in Samoa, as a way of suggesting ways of reading history from the body up. I have been arguing here for an approach to the body which recognizes its historical nature in two distinctive but inseparable ways, as both a function or condition of history in that large sense of cultural transformation at the macro level, and as a lived history or concourse of events, experience and reflection which makes up each individual life course as an idiosyncratic process.

There is a deep and occasionally divisive stress line in *Fa'a Samoa* between what Samoans refer to as tradition and what they call modern Samoa. This is a kind of exacerbating fracture which both energizes and destabilizes commonality and consensus. While certain core values, including the three I have focussed on in this book — dignity, humility, and strength — remain constant as the most abiding aspects of Samoan propriety and social order, their application and explication are subject to interested interpretation and deployment. Samoans themselves see this as a dispute between a desire to preserve some pure form of tradition and what proponents of the opposing view see as a more forward looking and accommodating modernity. Samoan history suggests that Samoans have in fact and action been remarkably accommodating, forward looking and open to social change, but Samoans

189

themselves have to an extent at least become arrayed into competing camps in which tradition as a fixed and stable historical code is engaged as either a positive moral end in itself, or as an obstacle to be overcome. As I said at the outset of this book, *Fa'a Samoa* is more like a path than a destination. This kind of future orientation is at the heart of *Fa'a Samoa*, and while the preservation and adherence to tradition may strike tourists, and some anthropologists, as conservative and hide bound, that mistakes rhetoric for motive. However, in practice today *Fa'a Samoa* is not just a cultural ideal, a formula for living, but is being manipulated politically in an increasing factionalization, both at the national and village levels, and is often engaged with as an object, a kind of statutory and inflexible framework which determines social action rather than only conditioning the range of possibility. This is more than a difference between culture as practice and culture as rhetorical design, and while *Fa'a Samoa* remains inherently supple in its ability to incorporate changes in conditions and ideas, the emergence in the social field of a more formal model of "good" vs "bad" Samoan culture has important implications for the future history of Samoa and the lives of Samoans. Some of these implications are being played out in realms of embodied practice itself. I have already mentioned some in earlier chapters. The institutionalization of the *fa'afafine* sex as a life long sexed and gendered position is one and the emergence of a discourse of sexualities which shifts the defining of sexed and gendered bodies inward to innate or essential states is another. The increasing reliance on over the counter drugs as a way of deflecting attention and social risk in disease, and the reliance on low nutrient but high status foods such as rice is another. I want, in this chapter, to expand on these in order to focus attention on the web of health related issues in which embodying practice is the key component, and through which an embodied perspective can provide insights into the causes and consequences of these changes.

Small is Beautiful: Dieting, Fasting, and the Thinning of Gender

In a ramshackle collection of small business buildings on the Fugalei Road, one of the three main roads running through the town area of Apia, there is a health club. Located on the second floor of an old wooden building, the club is made up of two rooms from each of which one can hear sibilant dance music most late afternoons. Inside, groups of women, mostly in their 20's and early 30's, and always accompanied by several *fa'afafine* run through routines of aerobic exercise. These women are distinctive in that they have body figures closer to those one finds in mainstream American and European fashion magazines than to what one most often sees on village roads throughout Samoa. They are thin, with the classic hour glass shape of fashion models and stand in contrast to the rounder, fuller, and more imposing shapes of most women their age. They are, in the words of one informant, "the *fa'afafine* ladies" because, she explained, they want to look like "those skinny fifty-fifties and not like real Samoans." Or, perhaps more compellingly, another woman dismissed them as "*palagi* girls, not Samoans at all." What this small group of women represents, and in the mid-1990's which is the last time I have reliable numbers, this club had slightly less than 200 members, is a trend which has been seen elsewhere in the Pacific as well [Becker 1995]. Small but slowly increasing numbers of women, and to a lesser extent, men, have adopted a rhetoric of dieting, exercise and body image drawn from mainstream overseas discourses of beauty as a way of expressing what many explained to me as a "modern" or "global" sense of identity and beauty.

Beauty is a key aspect of Samoan identity. Both men and women adorn themselves, with flowers or with brightly coloured clothes. It is not uncommon to encounter young men wearing make-up or nail-polish, for example. Unblemished skin should, Samoans will tell you, be framed by other beautiful things. But traditionally this beauty was also framed by size and slow and steady movement as the proper way of presenting ones body in the world. The good body was large, round, and carefully adorned. The women at the health club on the Fugalei Road are inverting this image almost completely. Their goal is something lithe, angular, and able to move quickly. Their gestures, even outside the health club setting, are sharper, quicker, and even their speech is more rapid. They eschew Samoan dress, whether the conventional *lavalava* or the more stately floor length dresses which have been the mainstay of older womens wardrobe since the turn of the century.

The emergence of a passion for dieting, even if only among a small group of women, is a fundamental change in Samoan body praxis which challenges basic Samoan notions of health and propriety in several ways. Dieting is about stopping the flow of food into and through the body, a restriction of the normal functioning of healthy bodies. While Samoans are adept at fasting, as their pattern of fast and feast in their eating habits shows, this fasting is directed outward as an expression of humility and strength, and as a way of enhancing dignity, since the ability to fast is evidence of an ability to do without and so to share. What the dieting women are expressing is the opposite of that altruistic version of the fast, since the goal in dieting is a specialness which overturns humility in favour of a distinctiveness in which the body is the core sign. Dieting is a setting apart rather than a joining together of individuals in which good health, the core value of restraint, and the day to day practices of sharing as a form of self indulgence are dismembered from the body of the family or community as a whole, and emerge instead as expressions of wilfulness and self expression. While concern over the health of these women was often raised, it was their immodest display of specialness and its implications that people most often commented on.

Indeed, most Samoans I know spoke with scorn about these women, the women wondering how anything so thin could ever expect to give birth and nurse a baby, and the men expressing something close to disgust at the idea of marrying someone so obviously ugly and irresponsible. While aerobic exercise can improve endurance, which is the basic feature of Samoan strength, these women, by virtue of their size alone, are considered weak.

For the women themselves, the goal is a mode of body practice which, in their very physical presence, defines them as modern. Success and accomplishment for them is something measured by their capacity for self-sacrifice, but the motivation of this sacrifice is self-actualization, not communal and familial partnership. What these women are engaging with their dieting and exercise is a model of self-interest, something self-centred rather than networked to other community concerns. These women exemplify the emergence of individualism in Samoa, an individualism being enacted through changes in their very bodies themselves. A recent study reported by Brewis et al. [1998] is suggestive of a wide spread shift in what these authors refer to as ideal body size, where they found that these ideals are indeed slimmer than the average body size of most Samoans, findings consistent with a similar trend in Fiji [Becker 1995]. However, it is unclear from their data if they actually controlled the concept of idea body size sufficiently to draw more than a very tentative conclusion that the dieting women are part of a larger trend. Samoans often say and then do quite contradictory things, at least to outside observers. To the question "what is the ideal body size" during my original fieldwork, both men and women would indicate something closer to the North American idea of thinness. But further probing on this question, asking about what they hoped to look like in the coming years, or about the healthiest body size, revealed that the thin ideal was expressing something distinctive that spoke more to ideas and ideals of modernity than it did to personal body preferences. My own data suggests that for most Samoans, the best body to have remains one which is large and strong, and that thinness remains deeply associated with illness, self-indulgence, and wrongdoing.

But even with that caveat, the thin-body ideal, as an ideal, is one which is ramifying outward to the villages throughout Samoa, with important health consequences. One area of young womens health which was raised over and over during my time in Samoa related to sudden weight loss in adolescent girls. While conventional illness models ascribed this most often to attack by malicious spirits, there was a sense among many of my informants that there was an emerging epidemic of these attacks and there was concern that the effect of this could undermine and destabilize Samoan families. Many saw quite clearly that the source of the attacks lay in young womens growing attachment of foreign models of beauty and gender, noting that these thinning young women were breaching modesty by striving to follow irresponsible models of attractiveness which renounced their responsibilities to their families and communities. The consequence was punishment by spirits, and a slow form of suicide in which the spirit became the agent.

There is a deep and difficult to penetrate sense of helplessness among family members confronted with this, because traditional methods of intervention either through healing treatments or appeasements to the spirits, have had quite uneven and not very long lasting results. Young girls recovered, only to fall victim to these attacks again, parents explaining that their attachment to these foreign models had not left them and they would continue to be punished, and even die, if they did not abandon these desires. The thinning girls were writing a different experience of gender, one which appeared to deny the central values of deference and obligation in favour of one which was individualized and innate and the conventional models of well-being and cure appear to have little or no comprehensive effect.

The insinuation of new body models is never simply a matter of aesthetics, but can carry with it an entire panoply of competing and conflicting values and ideas about other kinds of social relationships and this is certainly the case with the emergence in Samoa of a growing problem of anorexic behaviour by adolescent girls. While the health club women on the Fugalei Road are more often than not dismissed as an aberration by most Samoans, the wasting girls in the villages pose a more fundamental problem as they write a different order of gendering and sexing through their fasting. Their gendering praxis renders them beyond help, and for many Samoans, beyond hope because their actions deploy a body which is ultimately beyond the control of the communal order, disentangled and expressed as something fundamentally foreign. This foreignness isolates the dieting women because the conventional practices of embodiment no longer apply. Even the *aitu* are incapable of restoring orderliness, so much so that their intervention can lead to death itself. As such, dieting undermines a key way in which propriety and social order are embodied by undermining the authority of possession to punish and rehabilitate. Ruth, an instructor at the health club on the Fugalei Road, had been treated repeatedly for possession as a teenager, because of her dieting. Each successive treatment brought shorter and shorter periods of a return to a more traditional pattern of eating. Finally, during the fifth "cure" Ruth left her village and her immediate family and moved to Apia to live with some distant relatives. Here, in a network of surveillance and concerns for propriety which is more explicitly pluralistic, she began to teach other young women to diet and exercise, finally joining with several friends in teaching at the small health club. Dieting, for Ruth, had become an act of defiance against an embodying order through the enactment of a different kind of body which, when it fails as a moral entity, dies, but when it succeeds, as Ruth and the other women at the health club in Fugalei are succeeding, disentangles them from the conventional methods of social control and allows them to engage the world with a degree of independence, and I suggest, increasing authority. Where the conventional structures of embodiment and social control lack a strategy for alternative body styles other than illness, possession and punishment, the dieting women on the Fugalei Road are creating a new discourse of healthy bodies which can solve the dilemma of dieting adolescents, but in the process, creates a new embodiment of independence which challenges and will continue to transform the bodily practices of order, sociality, solidarity, and mutuality at the centre of Samoan embodiment.

Troublesome Minds: Mental Illness and Modern Bodies

A day like any other in Apia, driving Ruta into work at about 8:30 in the morning. When we pull up in front of the Toyota dealer, I notice a crowd formed at a corner where the two buildings meet. They are a very quiet crowd, which suggests they are not watching a fight. Ruta leaves and I drive slowly away. Its then that I notice there is a man sitting on the sidewalk, dressed in a very dirty shirt and *lavalava*. From this distance I cannot hear, but he appears to be speaking. I head back home for breakfast. Later in the day, walking along the beach road with Julie, we pass the same man sitting on the sidewalk across the road from the Nelson Library. This time there is no crowd around him but I notice a large group of people under the awning of the NPF building watching him and talking among themselves. This time I can hear that he is not talking, he is singing. It does not sound like any Samoan I have heard. In the meantime, Julie has noticed some coins on the ground and has picked them up. As we walk along I point out the man on the sidewalk, asking her what he is up to. She notices him for the first time and stops dead still.

"Oh no, I didn't see him there. This is probably money people have thrown to him. I shouldn't have picked it up. What do those people think of me?"

"What is he doing?"

"He's probably sick — sick in his mind. That's what he is doing. He is probably sick in his mind."

But we are walking off now very quickly, Julie obviously very embarrassed at picking up the money and at the sight of a mentally ill or somehow deranged person on the street of Apia, singing what appears to be gibberish while people toss money to him. After we check the mail, we have to walk along the Beach road again, and this time the man is surrounded by a group including many young teens in their school uniforms. They encircle the man, who is still sitting on the sidewalk. This time I leave Julie and wander over to try and see what is going on. From the outer rim of the group I can hear that he is singing again, only this time every so often people in the watching group laugh. It still does not sound very Samoan to me, something more like abadabadaba with occasionally a word or string that sounds like a word. It is usually at these "words" that people laugh. The man is sitting on the sidewalk, legs crossed. He is very dirty indeed. I can hardly make out the colour of his skin beneath the filth. His face is encrusted with dirt and dried stains of food. His eyes are very pale — the whites stained, the pupils wide and looking off above the heads of the people in front of him. His singing is quite soft, still a run of gibberish with the odd word thrown in. A repeating rising and falling figure, punctuated by words.

I catch the eye of an older woman, holding onto the hand of a very young child, who frowns and then smiles. Julie, noticing where I have gone, comes up beside me and watches for a few moments before touching me on the arm and pointing away from the crowd. As we walk away I notice the older woman walking away in the same direction as us. I walk directly over to her, walking along beside her and saying "talofa" as deferentially as I can. She stops walking and turns to face me.

"Sick man — very sick. Not good to see that, ahh?"

"But why are all the people watching him?"

"He sings bad words — uses bad words about things — and that makes people laugh."

"Should children be seeing this — school children. There were a lot of school children watching him, listening to him sing."

"Ahhh, they are worse — they hear these words then they say them to each other on the bus or on the road and then they laugh. It is not good but maybe it reminds them who says these words and then they will think about that."

"What do you think is wrong with that man?"

"His mind is sick, he has a sickness in his mind and maybe he has other sickness — maybe because he coughs many times when he sings — but in his mind he is very sick."

"Does no one look after him?"

"The doctors maybe? The family—his family—where are they today when your son is sick in the street and people are laughing at him. Maybe they laugh at his family, ahh."

"What will happen to him?"

"Die—who can feed him—he will die. Ahhh, this is a bad thing to see."

By this time we have reached Nelsons and she takes her child by the hand again and turns to leave. "*Tofa soifua*," she smiles, walking off. Julie has lagged behind and I turn to let her catch up. All the way home in the car she is very quiet. Just before we turn off the Vaitele road she turns to me and tells me "that is not something you should have to see, someone who is that alone here—here in Samoa—that alone that he must get money on the street like that. Sick people should not be on the street. This is like Canada."

Homelessness and mental illness seem to be the twin devils of urbanization in the Pacific, as elsewhere. In 1992 I knew of slightly more than 100 people living on the streets of Apia, disconnected from their families and scavenging for food and handouts as best they could. In recent years, friends and contacts in Samoa and New Zealand tell me this number is increasing slowly, and their observations are consistent with my own, noting that most of these homeless people appear to be mentally deranged in some way. While it is sheer political rhetoric in North America to insinuate all the homeless hear are mentally ill, it is apparent that mental illness is a major contributor to homelessness in Samoa.

As I described in earlier chapters, Samoan sociality is premised on mutuality and a strong dedication to sharing and communal responsibility. This system of inter and intra family obligation and sharing diffuses such things a poverty and natural disaster since, in the largest scheme of all, the nation, each individual member can not only rely on each other member, but has some measurable degree of responsibility to all other members as well. Such a system can sustain even profound economic or disastrous changes, and so, in the wake of Cyclone Val in 1991, there was a widespread effort to rebuild villages, and in particular schools, which relied on this network of mutual obligation and support. And yet an increasing number of people are becoming disconnected from this system of mutuality and obligation. While my initial reaction to this apparent conundrum was that perhaps the scope of inequities, and so of individual poverty or powerlessness for example, was being masked either intentionally by the people around me, or more likely, masked by my observers inability to see, I came to realize that something more fundamental was contributing, to the phenomenon of homelessness in Samoa.

At the heart of this is a change in the practice of embodiment itself. Most observers have noticed that Samoans do not experience mind, that is interior mental states, as something amenable to outside observation [see, for example, Clement 1974 or Shore 1977]. In the absence of direct action by an individual, interior states, motives, and conditions of the emotions, for example, are inscrutable. While each individual has these states and conditions, they are not knowable in themselves but only in their consequential effect in social action. The incorporation of a new illness category, *ma'i palagi* or European diseases, undermines that model because, among other things, it posits a set of interior conditions which are indeed scrutable, though only in the context of this other model of disease. Xray and ultra-sound, blood tests and the microscopic examination of urine or faeces, propose, though do not impose, a different model of the knowable body than that encompassed by Samoan biology itself and so open up a new range of interior conditions and even internal organs which were unknown, because they were unknowable, in the past.

In my discussions with Samoans about what I glibly am referring to as mental illness here, there was an interesting, though often not well articulated, distinction being drawn between the brain and the mind. The brain, for my informants, is an organ which can become overheated, or can lack for fluid sustenance, or can be injured by *aitu* hitting it or tearing at it. Like the stomach or the liver or the *to'ala*, this organ had a role to play in the flow of substances into, within, and out of the body. And like these other organs, its injury or impairment could have both physical and behavioural consequences. In contrast, they spoke of the mind as something much more amorphous and ambiguous, some expression of organic processes but something more than that. I noted earlier that in Samoan biology emotions reside in the gut, but it was never clear from my discussions with Samoans where, conventionally, thinking takes place. What was clear was that the brain was only some small component of that, though the overall imagining of mental process remains for me vague and underdeveloped, something which is consistent with the strong dispreference for even speculating about these processes by Samoans. Extreme mental illness, which from my layman's perspective appeared in the instances I am familiar with to be forms of schizophrenia or other dissociative disorders, pose a diagnostic problem for Samoans because they render the individual so completely helpless, and from their perspective, so troublesome because of their unpredictable behaviour. Not amenable to conventional curing, but carrying with them all the social costs associated with illness, extreme mental disease is one class of illness which has been most readily re-incorporated as *ma'i palagi*, reducing its social cost but at the same, diminishing social responsibility for care and treatment. These are European diseases, effecting a part of the body only Europeans can see and treat, the mind, and for all practical purposes, a family can be said to be absolved of responsibility for something over which they can exercise no practical control.

And so responsibility for the care and treatment of those with extreme forms of mental illness can fall to strangers, in particular an underfunded mental health association and the department of public health of the national government. This risks making Samoans sound backwards and uncaring, and if that is the response these pages suggest, I suggest you read them again. There is a reasonable cultural logic to this phenomenon which has nothing to do with failing to take responsibility but rather expresses, poignantly, how responsibility needs to be accounted for in an understanding of the models of body process within which illnesses occur. Social responsibility in Samoa is not some abstract value, some higher order of moral obligation to which all else is subsumed, but a fundamental aspect of embodiment. The mind, for Samoans, is a troublesome thing and dealing with it when it breaks down stretches the ability of their embodying practices to accommodate new ideas, an ability which is considerable but not without its limits.

HIV/AIDS: Sexing Disease

The response to the HIV/AIDS, on the other hand, exemplifies how readily and easily new ideas can become accommodated into Samoan embodiment, and points to one of the reasons AIDS has had the kind of negative effect culturally which we see in the West. I am referring to models of body substances and their valuation and their properties. HIV/AIDS is about poisoned blood and semen, after all. In particular, it renders semen a substance of great danger, something evil. In contexts where semen is a substance of power, its contamination can have dramatic consequences, not the least of which is imperiling the very nature of relationship between being male and being good, a core component in all patriarchal systems. While HIV/AIDS first emerged in North America, for example, amongst gay men whose status as males was conventionally negated, a core association emerged between semen and disease, an association which challenged the central foundation of male dominance. Indeed, in the first years of the AIDS epidemic in the U.S., most of the effort at imagining the disease and giving it its own cultural rhetoric involved trying to deflect attention away from its connection with semen by focussing on issues of race, and even, for a while, female sexuality as the main culprits. The early rhetorics of safe sex appealed to historic images of diseased women and racial miscegenation, subverting the more fundamental association with diseased semen and disabled maleness. A history of the failure and success of North American responses to AIDS, which remains to be written, will need to take account of this basic problem which so much AIDS rhetoric has sought to evade.

When I first arrived in Samoa on a cold Sunday evening in September of 1991, the first thing I saw as the plane taxied to the terminal at Faleolo Airport was a huge sign which read quite simply: WELCOME TO SAMOA: Please Help Us Keep AIDS Out. In 1991 HIV/AIDS was a foreign disease, of foreign origin, and maintaining the barriers between Samoans and foreigners was the basic preventative strategy. While many people I spoke with about HIV/AIDS had a clear understanding of transmission and so on, a very common belief was that Samoans could only become infected by contact with foreigner, effectively asserting that Samoans could not spread HIV/AIDS among themselves. In December of that year, Catholic nuns joined with *fa'afafine* and others in World AIDS Day events, distributing condoms and literature which focussed almost entirely on keeping HIV/AIDS out of Samoa by controlling intimate contact with foreigners. Beneath this however, two conflicting imaginings and embodyings of HIV/AIDS were circulating, one which parallelled the North American concern with the purity of male substances and the other which linked HIV/AIDS with the still underdeveloped notion of sexual orientations as embodied positionalities and life defining scripts.

As I noted in an earlier chapter, male and female substances, and in particular semen and blood, are not, in themselves, special or sacred or dangerous things. Their importance lies in what happens when they are combined. This is particularly true of semen, which, while embarrassing to talk about because it draws attention to the penis, is treated with the same nonchalance as we might treat saliva or tears, something to be wiped away when spilt. Semen has powerful potential, but only in its relationship with other body substances such as women's blood. As such, a disease discourse which renders semen dangerous, while not without consequences, does not attach to such higher order issues such as male identity since Samoan men do not define themselves in this way. But in tracing out the effects of HIV/AIDS on embodiment, I encountered echoes of the associating of maleness and semen which parallelled that found in North America. Many men spoke of how they felt like their power was being undermined by HIV/AIDS because it meant they could no longer father strong children. Being the father of a strong baby is important to most Samoan men, but in these mens experience, something more basic was being challenged and undermined. Where traditional male and female fertility is about the concourse between male and female substances, in these mens experience, the imperiling of their semen imperiled their sense of maleness itself. The rhetoric of HIV/AIDS as a poisoning of semen was creating, for these men, a prioritizing of body substances in which one — semen — was seen as being the more powerful and important of these substances. They would talk about how HIV/AIDS would destroy the Samoan family, would lead to women taking over Samoa, would end in the weakening and death of all Samoan men, and so on. All this, it should be stressed, within a discourse which said HIV/AIDS could not be transmitted from Samoans to other Samoans.

There appears to be, in these mens comments, a concern with issues of foreignness and of "racial" purity on the one hand, and with a growing sense of fixed sexes and genders on the other, two things which when taken together appear to be producing a hierarchy of embodied objects in Samoan body sense. The other discourse emerging around HIV/AIDS, that related to sexual orientations, is another piece of this puzzle.

Increasingly, HIV/AIDS has come to be associated for Samoans with *fa'afafine*. The initial connection between *fa'afafine* and HIV/AIDS was about foreigners, since *fa'afafine* were believed to be more likely to have sex with tourists and other visitors than would other Samoans. Indeed, many people would dismiss *fa'afafine* as a class as nothing more than prostitutes. But the *fa'afafine* themselves took a quite pro-active approach to HIV/AIDS, recognizing quite early that their own sexual practices, and in particular anal intercourse, put them at considerable risk. They formed groups which assisted the public health department in country wide education programs, and policed themselves as well, providing a support network for other *fa'afafine* and increasingly, other young people, in developing HIV/AIDS awareness. These activities have been effective and HIV prevalence rates in Samoa are remarkably low, barely registering in a country where many other STD's are endemic. But there has been a consequence of these group activities which connects with a growing concern for "true" maleness.

HIV/AIDS activism on the part of *fa'afafine* has had the effect of bureaucratizing and rationalizing their status as a third sex in a more fixed and less fluid way. Criticism by non-*fa'afafine* Samoans, who have castigated them as the cause of HIV/AIDS introduction into Samoa, and the sense of being at heightened risk of disease themselves, has created a community of interest among *fa'afafine* where none existed before. HIV/AIDS has made *fa'afafine* stand out as a more formal and more stable category and has given many of them an identity which effectively distinguishes them from the other sexes in Samoa. A fundamental consequence of HIV/AIDS activism in Samoa has been the emergence, though still in a very early form, of a discourse of fixed, innate, and life-long sexual orientations which, when coupled with the growing sense among many Samoan men about the prioritizing of maleness over other sexes and genders, is having the effect of stabilizing sexed and gendered bodies in Samoa in ways which invert the more fluid and transient conventions of gendering and sexing. While other popular global cultural influences, especially among the young, are also part of this ongoing emergence, HIV/AIDS connection with embodied praxis is reconstituting the Samoan body in an interesting direction, effectively doing in a few short years what nearly two centuries of Christianization and the pursuit of modernity has been unable to do. The ultimate effects of these changes remain to be played out.

Women and Health/Women as Health: Gendering Power

In a different but equally far reaching way, a "traditional" village structure long associated with women is contributing to changes in embodying practice by connecting health, political power, education, and social control in the operations of womens village health committees. Historically, women were responsible for such things as the maintenance of the church grounds, the cleanliness of the water supply, and the safe and healthy preparation and presentation of food, as well as for overall attention to the health of village members. While men also took part in all of these things, it was more often than not under the direction and supervision of women. Although the preparation of the *umu* or earth oven, remains the domain of young men, the overall concern for food and health has long been associated with women. The creation of national structures for the implementation and funding of projects and the maintenance of order has involved the creation of village level structures through which these directives, funds and other resources flow. Chief among these has been the institutionalization of women's committees, which in most villages have assumed responsibility for the implementation of public health programs, maintenance of the schools and the enforcement of attendance, as well as their traditional role in the production of status wealth such as fine mats and bark cloth, which are exchanged on ceremonial occasions. The womens committees combine longstanding roles related to wealth, cultural reproduction, and the distribution of power with a new role connecting village structures upwards to national processes. This is not a one way relationship, however.

The women's committees stand in a special space between the new structures of national administration and traditional structures of village life and as such, serve as an important conduit through which social change is enacted. But they do so not only as agents for national policies but also interpreters and formulators. That is, they do not simply implement policy on behalf of the national agenda, they actively create those policies either through resistance to national agenda, or through an interpretive role, taking these policies and giving them form in the village contexts. This is particularly true in matters of health. As I noted in the last chapter, health surveillance is an important aspect of the maintenance of social order, since illness is almost always about some social wrongdoing and always has consequences beyond the individual patient to his or her network of relatives and associates. The centrality of women in the implementation of health related projects locates women and their village committees at the most potent nexus of power in Samoan village life. The authority to watch, diagnosis, impugn and enforce rehabilitation which are at the heart of the illness process confers a degree of power on the womens village committees which no other village structure has, not even the *fono* which is the official body for deliberation and decision making in village life. As one woman put it, "the *matai* argue about what to do but the village committee decides what is done, and then it just does it." The effect of womens dominant role in health surveillance is the slow accretion of power into the hands of the womens committees. This institutionalizes health, and the maintenance of healthy bodies, most directly as a political project with national scale implications since it has inadvertently created a power site which can, at its most active, shape nationwide practice by determining how policy is enacted.

One effect of this is actually a violation of the principles of consensus which function in Samoan decision making, because the committee emerges as a site of power which, while driven internally by consensus, can actually elide the wishes of the larger community in pursuit of its own goals. That it is, the womens village committees no longer simply act with the other village members, but act on their behalf as well. And it is the experience of illness as community or society wide social peril which empowers this elision. The contradiction between a consensus driven form of social power and the institutionalization of a rational structure which can abrogate that consensus makes sense only if we take into account the embodying practices through which the ill body connects with the community and because of which the community, either in part or in the whole, has a wide ranging interest. So much is at stake in health, from the maintenance of morally appropriate citizens to the sustenance, protection, and control of all social relationships, that the contradiction evaporates. In the context of more and more institutionalized national structures, a deepening concern with the revitalization of tradition on the one hand and the pursuit of the modern on the other, and the transglobal health threats which include but go beyond HIV/AIDS, the emergence of the women's village committees as both the guardians and the arbiters of the good and proper body in Samoa makes both cultural and historical sense.

It is in both a cultural and historical sense in which the body plays a central role, and which has the potential to reshape political power in Samoa in unexpected directions. The womens committees, while they often reject national policy and reformulate it as it is being applied at the village level, nonetheless do not stand in a relationship of necessary antagonism to the nation as a political force. They see their role as ameliorating and improving the effects of national policy, and not as competing with national policy making. In contrast, the *fono* or council of *matai* operating in each village has been simultaneously empowered and weakened by its relationship with the nation state. It was absorbed into the colonial power structure, serving as an agent for colonial policy in which the *matai* were as often complicit and collaborative as they were antagonistic and resistant.[1] But a consequence of this connection is that the power of the *fono* becomes interwoven with political factionalism at the national level, and since independence the negotiation of allegiance and authority between groups of *matai* has created divisions which transgress traditional connections of family to family alliance. As such, though the processes of authority and power, driven by family consensus and so on, remain intact, the *fono* has become for many Samoans anachronistic and even unneccessary unneccessary, because it mirrors national level institutions and so presents a double burden.

In contrast, the women's committees were not treated with great seriousness by colonial administrators and so remained relatively independent of factional divisions at the national level. Their sphere of influence, most especially health and social propriety, were simply not taken seriously by administrators more interested in commercial and other resource exploitation. In the years since independence, national governments have tended to remain focussed on issues of economic development, literally leaving what I have argued here is the nub of social power in Samoa to local level structures. Since the surveillance and maintenance of embodied propriety is the foundation of power in Samoa, even if structures such as the *fono* with their formality and drama give the impression of being the real arbiters of power, the consequence of colonial, and now post-independence, national policy has been a formalizing and strengthening of women's power as the gatekeepers of embodied propriety and community health. The womens committees have become the site and the expression of social power as a daily process, a lived engagement between community and the individual, and while formal structures such as parliament and the *fono* play key roles in national discourses of power, at the level of everyday life women's traditional association with health and propriety has allowed them to emerge as an increasingly important national actor, enacting real social power from the village, and ultimately, from the body upward.

The effect of this has been that the womens committees are taking authority over more and more village matters, ranging from those long the province of these committees, such as health, to, in some villages the adjudication of criminal behaviour, the building of new schools, occasionally in direct defiance of national programs, and in at least one instance the complete abrogation of the authority of the *fono* by the women's committee. In this instance, the women took over all dealings with the national government, which led to banishment of several *matai* on the orders, quite extraordinarily, of the womens committee. In one truly extraordinary case of power shifting, a young *matai* has actually built his rise to power on collaboration with several womens committees. Currently the holder of two important *matai* titles, Charlie was given these titles in open defiance, by the womens committees, of the choice made by the families, and the *fono* involved. More unusual than this, the womens committee decision was subsequently ratified by the families.

At the core of this change lies the basic entailments of embodiment and order in Samoan society, entailments which have devolved increasingly to women. Although women were historically the most active in such areas as health and moral order, this was not a gendered function. Men had long been involved with the womens committees in the same way women were long involved with the *fono*, the more formal site of authority in Samoa. But the evolution of national level factionalism, the prioritizing of economic political concerns over the more quotidian interests in who is doing what, to whom, if you will, has institutionalized a gender division in social power which, while still fragmented and emergent, reflects once again an increasing rigidity and formal dividing of Samoan sociality. This is not simply a matter of modern versus traditional values, though this discourse of preservation and propriety is important. Something more critical appears to be happening, an instantiation of a new cognitive map of the body in Samoa which focuses on essences, on new rules of similarity, and on increasingly impermeable boundaries which foreclose and limit experience by writing it in advance as something which comes from within the body, rather than as something the body deploys in its enactment.

* * *

Taken together, these transformations, from among many, connect with an increasingly formalized and rigid set of values and rules which stand in contention with the fluidity and transience of *Fa'a Samoa*. An embodied perspective allows us to see how these changes are related, and how they each in their own way are part of a general direction in social change in Samoa, social change which is being enacted through the practices of embodiment which I have been discussing throughout this book. An embodied perspective allows us to unearth the kinds of perils and influences through which, and because of which, fundamental changes at the heart of the culture process occur, by showing how they are given flesh and substance not simply as things people think about the world, but as things people do with and to the worlds they make.

Sione stood at the doorway of the womens *fale*, watching a circle of younger women seated in the centre of the room weaving leaf mats, which would be distibruted at the funeral later that week. The conversation was animated but soft, as the women discussed a recent visit by a nurse from the Department of Public Health in Apia. A few weeks earlier, as part of a national nutrition program, a nurse had given a lecture to the women of the village on the importance of supplementing babies diets with higher quality protein, along with the staple of rice, which for most of the women with infants in this village, remained the food of choice. The women weaving the mats were concerned that feeding their children lower value, that is lower status food in place of rice could pose a health threat to them as they started to grow. Sione stood listening to this discussion for several minutes before stepping into the centre of the circle and sitting, cross legged, in front of the young women. She took up several fronds and began plaiting them into the outer edge of a new fine mat. She joined in the conversation, pointing out that feeding babies rice ran the risk of creating too much pride in their bodies, given the high status attached to rice as a boiled white food. Maybe, she mused, we could boil some tinned fish with the rice, make it darker and less like rice. The other women laughed at this, one suggesting they mix cocoa with the rice and make it even darker, less the boiled white food it really was.

"The nurse would never know" Sione laughed.

As I listened to them discussing what the nurse had told them, and how they were adapting the nurses information to their concerns with the health of their babies, I remembered the first time I had been asked to sit in with the women while they made fine mats and talked. It was an honour to be asked, and I harassed my host with questions about mats, mat decoration, the value of different sizes of mats. After patiently answering my questions for most of the morning, Sione, who had invited me to the womens *fale*, turned to me and handed me several fronds of leaf from the pile at her feet.

"Touch this, Douglass. You see, you don't understand. It is not the mats, Douglass, it is the weaving."

Chapter 10

Elusive Fragments: The Embodying of Theory and Praxis

A serpent swam a vertex to the sun
– On unpaced beaches leaned its tongue and
    drummed.
What fountains did I hear? what icy speeches?
Memory, committed to the page, had broke.

"Passage"
Hart Crane

During the first week of my stay in Samoa, I became ill from drinking untreated water. I spent several painful days vomiting and passing out before my body finally accustomed itself to the organisms present in the water. This experience, so early in my fieldwork, had important consequences for the direction I have taken in this text. When, during those first few days, I lay sick in my house, I was being drawn into a set of practices which rendered my body unknowable by the standards I had brought along with my notebooks and computer and questions. When Pai, my late Samoan mother, brought me undercooked eggs and tea to treat my nausea, she was initiating me, without knowing it, into a spiralling confusion about what something as simple as curing a stomach ache could mean for understanding culture.

Of course, I did not know that at the time either. As I lay there wondering when I would vomit again, I knew exactly what was going on. I knew what Pai's eyes meant when they twinkled at the news my bowels were once again working, and I knew what the tea and sugar was for. I understood why Sene, my ten-year-old Samoan "brother," kept asking me if I was sad. It was only later, as I reflected on those long days, and what my Samoan friends had told me about their own bodies, that I realized everything I thought I knew was either insufficient or wrongheaded. The pain, interests, and care I had experienced were veiled by a way of relating to my body, and to my experiences, which was often completely at odds with what those around me were doing to my body and what they assumed I was

207

experiencing. It was not simply a matter of having different information, or even different expectations, which was certainly true enough. What I came to realize was that we had different kinds of bodies altogether. The very nature of the body my family and friends were watching and treating was different from the body I was allowing to be watched and cared for. We were both bodies in the world, but we were in the world in different ways.

Later, Charlie would sit with me at night, answering my questions, and probing my reasons for asking them, making me rethink them even as I put them to him. Then he would simply stop me short and ask me why, if I really wanted to know, I didn't just do it. He was being practical. It all made sense to him, from the strengthening I would experience if my mother had taken me to be circumcised as a boy, to the dignity I received and expressed each time I ate the guest's portion of a pig at a formal meal or *fa'alavelave*. I took a long time to understand that asking questions about Charlie's acts of intimacy and friendship toward me removed me from understanding that when he lay his head on my lap and told me filthy jokes about pigs and the minister's wife, he was engaging me and my body in a web of connection, support and meaning. It is that web of contact and complicity that I have navigated here.

Intimacy, participation, and collaboration: those are the things I was being initiated into with Pai's painful cure of for my nausea, or Charlie massaging my foot when I told him that sandals made my toes hurt. My body made perfect sense to them. It took me a lot longer. For a long time my body was engaged in a kind of conquest, trying to render down and contain the bodies around me with a common sense that did not fit. In the process of being engaged as a meaningful body by the Samoans I lived and worked with, I was being enticed into a different order of sense, pleasure, and obligation. I was being made to see, feel, and understand my own body in a different way. My argument in this book has been an attempt describe how this difference is accomplished in the practices Samoan's use to create their bodies in the world. The complicit presence of my own body can never be isolated from the processes of Samoan embodiment I have been describing.

In writing the ethnography of Samoan bodies I have presented here, I have constructed what Boddy refers to as "a kind of allegory based...on actual observations of human foreigners, but...put together to meet the demands for cultural coherence which 'the author' shares with [his or her] audience" [Boddy 1989:357]. I have not represented Samoan bodies, so much as I have described how those bodies are a process of representation, accounting, and experience. In a sense, I have analyzed Samoan bodies into existence as a metaphor for the process of embodiment Samoans themselves are engaged in. This text is a metaphorical speculation on how

Samoans come to have and sustain meaningful bodies in the world, and a speculation on how these practices can be described and theorized.

In these remaining pages, I want to draw together some of the themes which have emerged in my descriptions and reflections on Samoan practices of embodiment in order to outline the preliminary framework for a model of embodiment, culture and being.

Finding the Body: A Summary of Issues and Themes

At the outset of this book, I outlined what I see as the major problem with previous attempts to theorize the body. In most cases, these efforts have treated the body solely as something which is acted upon by forces of culture. As I argued there the problem with such approaches are that they leave unexamined the question of how, and under what conditions, the body comes to be meaningful at all. The body, in these approaches, is just another object to be manipulated by culture, ignoring the more basic issue of how objects are made to be present in the world.

I argue that a model of embodiment must take as its focus the process of generating a meaningful body through action, as one of the central practices by which culture is enabled and enacted. It combines the formulae "culture makes bodies" and "bodies make culture" into a single tautology: making bodies is about making culture which is about making bodies. It is this combination of processes, practices, and effects which needs to be addressed in the continued development of such a model, because the body is always a basic and unavoidable aspect of culture and action. Through this concatenation of processes, effects, structures, and influences, we can approach the body as a "memoir born of the dialectic between what is given to us and what we make of it" [Jackson 1989:18, citing Nietzsche].

This parallels Stoller's comments, where he argues that studies of the body, such as Featherstone et al. [1991], with their consideration of such subjects as

> diet, appetite, consumer culture, martial arts, aging, and human emotions...are topics worthy of embodied reformulation... [but they] do not take us much beyond the body-as-text, a metaphor that strips the body of its smells, tastes, texture and pain [1994:637].

Culture, I am suggesting, is not a story told about the body. Rather, it is a story told through, with and because of the body. More importantly, it is a story we tell because of the kinds of bodies we come to have as participants in the active process of constituting the cultured world around us. With Stoller, I argue for rigorous, critical attention to the cultural limits on body sensation, and the culture generating effect of sensation itself. Whether the taste of food, the flash of embarrassment when a brother sees his sister bathing, or the emotional contentment a *matai* feels when he takes his portion of the pig at a formal meal, I argue that moving beyond the limitations of previous approaches to the body needs to take into account that crucial circular relationship between the body and culture which

> governs all forms of incorporation, choosing and modifying everything that the body ingests and digests and assimilates, physiologically and psychologically [Bourdieu 1984:190, cited in Stoller 1994:637].

It is this relationship of interpenetrating cause and effect which demands a model of the body that moves beyond its simple narrative aspects, as one of the many stories culture tells, by siting the body as a sensual centre, in and through which culture is experienced and enacted.

Let me review some of the ground of embodiment in Samoan body practice, but with a reassertion of a key point which has run through this text. Is what I have been describing here nothing more than a catalogue of socializing effects, a set of learned responses which members of a society incorporate in the sense of wiring them unwittingly into their flesh? In the preceding chapters I have assiduously avoided the word "belief," because I feel the concept of belief dichotomizes knowledge into truth and reality, and obscures the active process of knowing through which the world is rendered sensible. Belief is a judgement of truth, and a test of reliability and value. It may or may not direct or determine action, and it is always a wilful act of evaluation. Knowing, on the other hand, is an understanding, that is, a direct engagement with the world, that experiences and explains it simultaneously. While it is possible to no longer believe something, as in no longer believing in the tooth fairy, it is never possible to "un-know" something. Once understood, the world is inexorably different from what it was, and even as understandings shift and change, the effect of understanding is always the same. The world is, inextricably, what we know it to be. We can never not know something we have known. My argument in this text has not been an argument about beliefs, but about understanding and knowledge. Samoans do not "believe" in the *to'ala*, they experience and know it. They do not believe that space is ranked according to a measure of dignity and visibility, they experience it as such. Each time they walk or talk, they are enacting this knowledge. To call this "belief" is dismissive and ethnocentric in the extreme. There is no test of truth against which knowing can be measured, because knowing is not about truth. It is about being, and being sensible, in a world we make sensible by knowing it.

An example might illustrate this more clearly. In the final movement of Beethoven's Waldstein Sonata, the main theme is restated in the final pages, played in double time. The physical act of playing this many notes is demanding and complex. It involves the pianist "wiring in" through practice, the necessary movements of her hands, because were she to "think" about the moves required, she would not be able to play the notes at their proper speed. At the same time, she has incorporated into her "wired in" ability to play these passages, assessments of an aesthetic, expressive nature. She performs the sonata, not simply as a series of fast manipulations of piano keys, but as an expressive act. The sonata has become embodied, in the sense of being experienced, through the body of the pianist. She does not believe in the movements needed to make the expressive statement she will make when she performs this piece. She knows it, incorporating an understanding of the aural dynamics of the concert piano, and the synœsthesic relationships between sound, emotion, and touch, into the deployment of her posture, and the movement and pressure of her fingers. She becomes the sonata in a truly embodied form.

The element of learning, either of the Waldstein Sonata, or the proper way to weave a pandanus leaf mat, is essential to understand how anyone can, physically, do such things. However, understanding that learning process is not the complete story. Living the act of playing a Beethoven sonata, as an enactment of an embodied experience of the world, needs to be scrutinized as much as the training which makes it possible. Every move of the *fofō*'s fingers in examining a feverish child, or children playing in and around their houses in a Samoan village, I have been arguing, is an act of socializing the world by deploying a socialized body in it.

The Body Encountered

The bodies of infants and strangers are problem bodies, because in the instant of their acknowledgement, they need to be recognized and codified for what they are, and how we can reasonably anticipate they will behave. In the process of pregnancy and infant recognition Samoans begin a lifelong practice of attending to the body, which not only realizes the expectations of meaning which can be nominally attached to any body, but instructs the newly observed body in the precepts of appropriate deployment through which it will enact itself in the world. We saw in Chapter

4, for example that certain basic notions about body substances, and their proper presence in the world, are embodied in the acts of sex, foetal development, and in the treatment of the newly born infant, as it stumbles and cries under the constant attention of caregivers and onlookers. The developmental nature of the body, as something moving toward restraint and modesty as it achieves its final social form, is encoded in the treatment of the mother during pregnancy, with rules and concerns about protecting her own body in order to protect the final form of the child's body, and in infancy with the tolerance of noise, constant eating, and uncontrollable bowels, which characterize the first months of life.

At stake in these first efforts of attention is the laying of a ground of meanings within which the child can engage the world as a participant rather than a particle. Understanding the nature of body form and function direct the treatment of the child. As the child moves into its own space of awareness and complicity in embodied sociality, it does so with knowledge of the limits and expectations of the world around it, and the people with whom it connects. This "preobjective" knowledge becomes the ground of engagement from which the child emerges, slowly, as fully human, and fully connected, in the co-operative mosaic of bodies conjoined in mutual construction. The combinations of semen and blood, the forcing of substances into and out of the infant's body, the way the child is held and manipulated in games and in caregiving, and the constant drawing of the child's attention to the enacted world around it, outline the limits of how that world can be known, and gradually direct the infant toward knowing the world, and their meaningful place in it.

The Body Enlightened

In the acts of learning the limits of appropriate space, and the bodies which can be deployed in the different kinds of space in which the Samoan child moves, a different process is slowly enacted. It is one which begins to define the world through the physical act of the child's body moving in it. Socialization connects lived space with body substances, manners of movement and noise, ways of seeing and being seen, and the dangers and comforts which culture attaches to space. The world in which the child moves becomes a world incorporated, that is, a world that contains his or her understanding and experience of modesty and humility, obligation and responsibility, and good and bad. In the socialization of lived space in Samoa, the basic concept of *lēaga*, socially bad or dangerous, becomes part of the child's very experience of its body as it moves through daily life.

I deliberately chose the word enlightened in beginning this section. In this process of incorporation through which the child becomes a formal and knowledgeable participant in the embodiments of everyday life, Samoans have a deep concern with the space of light, and the space of darkness. Enlightened space is the space of community, visibility, and co-operation, while the space of darkness is the space beyond the illumination of society, where individuals pursue individual desires and concerns. The child learns a fear of the dark in both a physical and metaphorical sense. It is a fear that is enacted by the ways the child comes to deploy its body. Physically, the child learns the dark is the space of dangers, either from *aitu,* or from paths that become obscured in the darkness. It is the space of monsters, in a very real and physical sense. The child also learns that the dark is a space which puts at risk the very nature of who he or she is as an embodied person in Samoan society. To be out of view and hidden, and especially to purposefully seek invisibility, become laden with fear and concern. The child learns to seek the comfort of the light in the centre of the village. In this sense, the dark space outside of sociality becomes a persistent space of initiation and re-initiation. In its movement back and forth over these boundaries, the child comes to enact the embodied space which makes its body possible.

The Body Enraptured

Play and work are two sites at which the full force of the process of embodiment is engaged in the life of any society. In play and work, the body is expressive and exploratory, extending itself wilfully into the world around it. Doing and being in the world are inseparable, connected in a single process of embodiment. Having a meaningful body structures and manipulates the world by incorporating the world into the body itself.

In Samoan play and work, the world becomes a coded place of appropriate connections between pleasure and sociality. It is in work and play, from the complex acts of building a house, to the simplest act of a child playing under a tree during a rain storm, that the body sustains itself as a presence in the world. The village centre becomes the place of intersubjective play and cooperation, while solitary play is reserved for the a-social periphery.

In work, and in play, and in this we need to include marital sex and sexual play, Samoans learn the need for the darkened periphery. They engage it in their individual pursuits, but they do so with an eye on the light they are leaving behind. The enactment of bodies in work, and in play, enacts the obligations of sociality and individuality in the demarcation of space that bodies doing different things embody in different ways. The child playing alone with his truck on an isolated village road, teenagers courting under bushes in the night, or boys working in solitude to clear away the weeds in the taro patch, are each embodying space with the manner in which they deploy their bodies, both in labour and pleasure. In the same way, brothers and sisters joking or dancing, husbands and wives eating together and discussing the day's events, or children inviting each other to share in their toys or their bags of potato crisps are deploying social space in the manners of their embodiments.

The body in work and play explodes the social field with its variations and simultaneous return to order and stateliness as it moves in and around the boundaries of the world that its actions create. The body of the playing child, the bodies of boys fighting along the darkened roads at night, or the bodies of *matai* deep in conversation over their morning tea, are each engaged in a similar process, however diverse the activities they pursue. They are making spaces within which the various expressions of the good and proper body can be deployed, by deploying their good and proper bodies within them.

The Body Encompassed

Discipline is never isolated from the body in rapturous deployment in the acts of working and playing. Indeed, discipline is always the energizing core of even the most mundane act of pleasure or labour in Samoa. Whether the inherent embodiment of discipline in the deployment of appropriate space, or the formal discipline of the arrangement of *matai*'s bodies in the *fono*, discipline and surveillance are fundamental to Samoan sociality. So basic is the pervasiveness of discipline and surveillance, that even in the darkest private spaces, where the necessary pursuits of individual bodies are encouraged, social forces in the form of *aitu* and ancestors, and the bodies deployed there themselves, extend surveillance and social control, so that nothing is ever completely invisible or hidden.

Discipline is about stillness, modesty, and quiet propriety. Acts of discipline, such as the arrangement of ranked bodies in the *fono*, the punishment and violence through which rules are enforced, and the way bodies become silent as they move through the spaces of dignity with which the body maps the world, have the effect of incorporating and reincorporating bodies and acts into the still order of the communal whole. When a child is beaten, or when the paramount *tulafale* calls out the house positions of the *matai* at a *fono*, the bodies engaged are not being marked as special or isolated bodies, but as the necessary bodies of orderly stillness which is the dignified centre of *Fa'a Samoa*. The disciplined body in Samoa is not a docile one. It is an instigator which enacts in its deployments the topography of propriety through which the Samoan body is experienced.

The Body Endangered

And then people fall sick. In discussing illness and healing, my primary concern was with the principles of connection between ill bodies and the world around them, and with the processes of illness which define bodies out of step, and seek to draw them back toward incorporation in the embodied sociality of the community. At stake in illness in Samoa, is the integrity of the enacted body, because illness endangers one of the most important sites of culture. Illness in Samoa also makes the body dangerous, because illness is never self-limiting, but always implicates those around the ill person. It enacts the co-operative core of Samoan sociality, and also engages the body in constant surveillance. Illness endangers propriety and dignity, not only for the body of the ill person, but for the socially meaningful bodies of those around it. Treating a headache becomes an act of restoring or sustaining dignity, as much as the formal speeches and exchanges at funerals or weddings.

Illness also illuminates and reinforces the experience of knowing which Samoans bring to bear on the world they live in. Processes of diagnosis and treatment, in restoring the orderly geography of the organs, the proper flow of substances into and out of the body, and the restraint on presence embodied in posture and motion, restate, in practice, fundamental understandings of the dignified nature of the social world. This enactment of dignity, whether in the movement of the bowels or the strength of muscles or the proper consistency of semen, renders dignity inseparable from the lived experience of the body.

The ill body is a body engaged by processes of discipline in the same way as the body of the disobedient *matai* trussed like a pig and left on the *malae* to be ridiculed and reviled. Each in their own way endanger the community. Silence and stillness surround healing as the community watches its own slow restoration. So much is at stake in illness, that the world almost stops, held in abeyance until the healthy, reconnected, proper body returns. That Samoan diagnosis and healing is often simple and undramatic should not obscure the fact that, in the watchful eyes of the family and village as the *fofō* negotiates the diagnosis and outlines a cure, the most basic of fears about the dissolution of society are being expressed and monitored. Illness is the discipline of society as a whole, enacted in the body full of fevers or covered in sores or vomiting grey bile and blood.

The Enchanted Body/Bodies
That Enchant The World

The Samoan body is an intricate mask, and a complex of masquerades, through which it manoeuvres around tensions and ambiguities in the social landscape. Bodies are special things, special processes, and each one is distinctive, each one has its own commands and demands on and within the life of the community. Submission and authority conjoin in the same body. Restraint and excess balance themselves on individual bodies, on each action, each step or gesture a body makes in and on the world. As such, the body is a kind of crisis of objectification. It stands for itself, as itself, and as other things, simultaneous with the experience of its existence by the consciousness it encompasses. Consciousnesses it encompass, since the body can never be said to exist except when it is engaged by the bodies around it. The body is restless, immaterial, and fleeting, mindful of itself while, at the same, profoundly forgetful of its constructed nature and social being. The body, I have been suggesting here, poses a fundamental conundrum which is the source of cultures most intimate energy.

Mindful and troublesome, fixed and persistently ambiguous. And so a masquerade. Samoans entangle their living bodies in a skein of masks and impersonations, as one way of fixing the illusory body and deflecting the tensions these bodies create. Uniforms, whether the school uniforms of children, or the uniform the *taupou* puts on as part of the process of enacting a formal meeting of *matai* each create similarity and specialness as a way of negotiating the competition of demands and desires which circulate in everyday Samoan life. The *fale aitu*, with their elaborate costumes and ribald inversions of submission and power create a space where the body, as a kind of effect of ambient light on the social field, can be stepped back from and, to the extent such a thing is possible, neutralized and made momentarily safe. *Fa'afafine*, with their blurring of the constraints of biology, energize flexibility and make ambiguity a virtue, keeping the flow and flux of the body as the sign of something happening, from freezing into some barbarous imprisonment where the body is rendered pure, static, and lifeless. An element of disguise helps Samoans manage the elements of surprise which overpopulate their daily lives with obligation and constraint, excess and sensuality, by making the body an enchanted thing which enchants the world it makes and moves in with possibility rather than prosecution.

Taken together, illness, tattooing, socialization, and the formal and informal enactments of proper bodies, express and create the key values of order and restraint, which characterize and energize *Fa'a Samoa*. Throughout their lives, Samoans pursue a physical presence which enables them to participate in the world as meaningful, and suitable bodies. Figure 9.1 illustrates this. The body, imagined into social presence through the linked practices I have been calling embodiment, is at one and the same time, an organic, objective reality, and a transient, culturally and experientially specific effect. When Jerry, a neighbour in Vaimoso, came out of his house the morning after Cyclone Val had finally moved away from the islands, and danced quietly in the mud which had trapped the family truck, he was engaging in a dance that connected him to the meanings, restraints, and expectations which centred his body in the world. His dance expressed, in its grace and delicacy, a tentative but expansive joy. It was an act of memory, and projection, in which the experiences of the previous five days were contained and completed, in a poised reassertion of his commanding presence as a body which enacts the world by being, meaningfully, in it.

The Paths That Bodies Take into the Light

I have argued, throughout this text, for a model of the body which connects each of these complicit, and interpenetrating, practices—learning appropriate space, and the appropriate kinds of bodies that can be present there: practices of discipline, submission, and surveillance, through which bodies are formed and sustained in daily action: the practices through which the healthy and the ill body are understood, recognized, and manipulated, not only in the prevention or treatment of illness, but in the observation of, and enactment, of good and proper bodies. Too often, the various sites of body manipulation have been treated in isolation, as limited practices. What this produces is a fragmented picture of the body as a set of discrete processes, losing sight of the lived quality of making bodies meaningful. What I have been arguing is that a critical model of the body as culture needs to explore the interconnections between these sites, as part of single process of being and doing a body. What I have been suggesting is a shift in the ground of body studies, from the exotic bodies of ritual, to the everyday bodies through which ritual is performed. Instead of a study of how institutions effect bodies, I have been arguing for a study of how bodies make institutions possible.

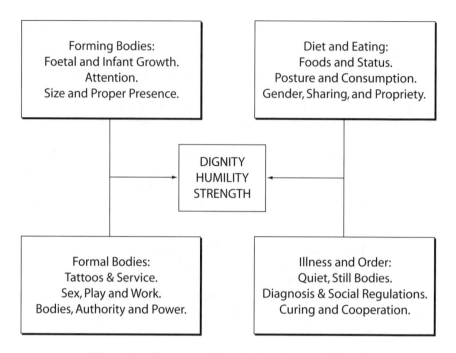

Figure 10.1 Summary of Associations between Cultural
Ideals and Embodying Practices in Samoa.

What I am proposing builds on accomplishments in other areas of body study, both within anthropology, and without. Recent advances in medical anthropology, such as Scheper-Hughes and Lock's [1987] argument for a more critical approach to the combination of bodily practices within which illness is practised, in the anthropology of the body, such as Csordas's [1994] model of knowledge of body experience as a preobjective field of meaning which determines the possible meanings, and consequences, body experience can have in a particular culture, have opened up new areas of description and analysis in body study. I have been exploring some of those areas and issues, in the context of a discussion of linked embodying practices in Samoa. I began my own study of Samoan embodiment, because of a dissatisfaction with the position of the body in anthropology. The body as an ongoing, lived, experience has been under-theorized in Anthropology. My argument, building on works such as those discussed in Chapter 2, which explore a parallel dissatisfaction with the way the problem of the body has been addressed in anthropology, has suggested one possible direction a renewed interest in the body might take. The body has never been too far from the surface in anthropological studies, but its presence has been too long taken for granted. What I, and those others whose I have described, argue for, is a critical re-evaluation of the relationship between culture, making sense of the body, and making sensible the world which both the body and culture occupy. That the body is, and should be, a fundamental focus of anthropological study, is not in itself a new idea, as the range of body studies I discussed in earlier in this book demonstrates. What is new, and I believe implicates a paradigmatic shift in the focus of the anthropological study of the body, is the recognition that in the intimate, everyday practices of embodiment such as those I have described here, culture is understood, constituted, and expressed. Walking and talking, I am arguing, are no less important to sustaining culture, and creating lived history, than the imposition of orders of slavery or the enactment of ritual secrets. By shifting the focus away from special bodies, toward an approach to the body which centres on the most mundane of quotidian activities, I am arguing for an anthropology of the body which is no longer a special kind of anthropology. I am suggesting that whatever the focus of study anthropologists choose, approaching it through how, and to what effect, the body is implicated, can add insights, and new kinds of knowledge and understanding. To repeat a point I have made repeatedly in this book, what I am suggesting is an anthropology which approaches culture and society from the body up.

Throughout this text, I have been raising issues of how the body is meaningful in Samoa in order to draw your attention to some of the key components I believe such a model of embodiment needs to address. I want to list some basic propositions around which I feel future work on embodiment should focus. I advance these propositions as a summary of the issues that the descriptions in previous chapters have raised, and as points of departure for future work in the field of embodiment study. They follow from one basic recognition I have been arguing for in this text: that self, personhood, identity, social structure, culture, and history, are inextricably linked to, and enacted by the body's presence in the world.

These propositions are ranked in the order of priority suggested by my descriptions and analysis of Samoan bodies in this text. However, the study of embodiment remains fragmented and incomplete, and this prioritizing of issues is preliminary and specific to the case I have been discussing here.

1. The body is not a thing, but a series of actions, guided by precepts and anticipations. It comes into meaningful existence through its enactment.

Any approach to embodiment must begin with what is done with the lived body itself rather than with an abstract, a priori, body of organic qualities, since even the organic nature of the body is subsumed by the practice of embodiment rather than the other way around. Embodiment does not respond to organic nature, but creates it. Unravelling the generation of anticipations and understandings of body function and form requires that the most fundamental components of the body, its organs and sensations, not be over-read as prior to experience, but be understood as aspects of experience itself. Body parts, that is, are cultural phenomena, and not simply the accumulated consequences of biology and evolution. As such, expectations about the body are a form of body knowledge inseparable from the experience of the body in specific circumstances and under specific constraints and conditions.

2. The body creates itself in its deployment rather than creating itself in order to be deployed. That is, the body is not simply a learned invented object, but a process of deployment which collapses object and action distinctions.

The body moves in space as a process rather than as a thing, insofar as movement is governed by the culturing action of making the body meaningful and moveable. In this way, the body is never actually fully present in space because it is always being re-formulated in its deployment depending on the obligations, exigencies, and vagaries of its encounters with other objects. Understanding the body as a path rather than a destination clarifies the complex relationship between being and time, because it allows us to think of the body in terms of emergence rather than objectification. The enacted body is just that, a performance of itself.

3. The deployment of bodies is both determined by the meaning of space, and an act through which space is made meaningful.

A conundrum any theory of embodiment will need to address is the fact that neither the body nor space can be said to be prior to the other. Although it is possible to speak of the constraints space imposes on deployment, and of the meanings deployed bodies enact on space, the direction of causation in this relationship is circular. The body makes space, which makes bodies, which make space, in a constant re-enactment of each other which cannot be accommodated by conventional models of causality or intention.

4. There are no properties of the body which are self-evident and universal in any, but the most mundane sense of being.

The sexing of bodies exemplifies this issue. Bodies appear, universally, to be of two forms, that is, male and female. Other sexed deployments are read as variations on this given attribute. In contrast, I am proposing, along with Butler [1993], that sexing itself be problematized as being a function of enactment rather than organic pre-determination. This does not mean male and female bodies do not exist, but that their experience as bodies is a function of embodiment rather than biology. Genitals are non-existent until practiced into existence as aspects of a deployed body, and as such, need to be read from their effects, rather than from their form. That is, like bowels or arms or eyes, they are not solely organic structures, but focal points of practices which invent them as body parts. A study of embodiment needs to address how this process is enacted, and what relationships it bears to such issues as ideology, roles, and power.

5. The body is an act of attention, and attention may take different forms, not only between cultures, but within them.

Attention refers not only to what can be seen, but also the manner in which things are seeable. Attention can focus on conformative similarity, digressive multiple meanings of single objects, or on the transgressive qualities of enacting objects in relationship to circumstantial exigencies. The practice of attention is a function of both individual recollections of cultural history, and the lived experiences of each body connected with other bodies in the historical field of a given society. However, defining attention as prior to the person attending to something is problematic, because it suggests an attending gaze beyond the body. This issue of where attention resides in social action needs to be explored more fully, in order to grasp how rules of seeing effect embodiment, as well as how the practice of embodiment effects the generation of rules of seeing. That is, the issue is not that all societies have rules of meaning. Rather, the issue is how those rules are embodied and transformed.

6. The body is not only an object of discipline, it is an act of disciplining the world in which the experience of the body colludes with expectations

of order and propriety to generate a good and proper universe.

I have stressed throughout this text that the bodies deployed in daily life in Samoa are co-participants in the structures of visibility and discipline which establish meanings and limitations on experience. The experience of discipline is not an imposition of docility on a waiting body, but an engagement between the world as thought about. and the world as experienced. This is another tautological relationship which needs to be exploded through more detailed analysis and consideration, because the issue of disciplined bodies penetrates all acts of embodiment, and makes embodied action possible. Excavating the disciplining effects of embodiment, as I have attempted here, is something a model of embodiment needs to pursue.

7. The body is not only thought about. Whatever the degree of rationalized distance with which we engage our body or its aspects, thinking about the body can never be extricated from the experience of our body, through which thinking is made possible.

The vast and complex literature of body image psychology [Fisher 1986] illustrates the complications of psychological approaches to the body, and to body awareness, drawing attention to a singularly difficult issue in embodiment. The act of thinking can never be isolated from the fact the body is a construction, a thing enacted through attention and awareness. Bodies and thinking about bodies are coterminous in the enactment of the embodied world, and must be deciphered in their connections, rather than dis-integrated into singularities. We do not so much think with the body as we embody the act of thinking.

8.A model of embodiment should have as its initiating impulse a determination to dismantle, or at least destabilize, conventional approaches to society and culture, which have obscured the lived enactments of the body.

Assertions such as "the body is not an object" or "the body is not something we do things to," or "the body is what we think it is," may seem to run opposite to what we intuitively know to be true. What I am suggesting here is that intuition is perhaps the compliment we pay to our biases. A model of embodiment needs to decentre intuition if it is going to get beyond the limiting expectations within which our own self evident bodies surrounds us. Earlier I quoted a student who suggested that the best definition of culture is that "culture is the act of creating culture." This is, for me, an insight which we should not lose sight of, in thinking of ways to approach and understand the body. What a model of embodiment needs to accomplish is the deconstruction of the comfort each of us feels in the body we know. A model of embodiment needs to make the bodies we are, that is, the bodies we bring to bear on the study of the body, problems in themselves. By subverting our own bodies, as practical enactments of a too taken for granted common sense, a model of embodiment can use the energy of our discomfiture to begin to unravel the possibilities for understanding the embodying experiences of others.

9. The study of the body, like the body itself, is inescapably fragmented, de-totalized, and frustrating. It is always only a beginning.

These are working propositions for a continued exploration of the practices of embodiment as a process of culturing the world. They are suggestive and tentative aspects of embodiment, which I have drawn from the ethnographic account of the Samoan bodies I have developed in this text. They point to questions which future research on the body as a comprehensive practice, may explore. For example, how do embodying practices change over time? If actual bodies, and ideas about bodies, are mutually determinative, what can produce changes in these practices? Are their modes of embodiment based, for example, on excess and restraint? I have noted that Samoan's do not have a semen conservation complex such as those found in Papua New Guinea. Does this suggest that for at least some peoples in Papua New Guinea, embodiment is governed by a model of the body which is defined in terms of the preservation and control of body substances, and if so, can analyzing these models tell us anything about these societies as a whole?

The link between embodiment and identity, such as the appropriation of tattooing by younger Samoans as an expression of an emerging ethnic identity, suggests other issues which a comprehensive study of embodiment may explore. What, for example, is the relationship between ethnic, racial, or national identity and the experience of good and bad bodies? In what way do ideologies of identity effect how the body is understood and manipulated? This area of body study over the last decade has been both substantial and innovative. It is an area on which the development of a critical model of embodiment can continue to build. For example, can the work of Parker et al. [1992], or Mosse [1985], on the link between nationalism, morality, political power, and ideologies of sexual identities, be extended to other areas of connection between the experience of the body and the practices of personhood? Can Taussig's [1987] analysis of the embodying effects of slavery in South America, or Comaroff's [1985] discussion of the historical links between Christianity, racism, and illness, among the Tshidi of Southern Africa, be developed further, as a way of approaching the question of how personhood, not only in extreme forms, but in all its forms, is deployed by, and through, the experience of the body? Can we take Feldman's [1991] argument that the civil war in Northern Ireland has created special kinds of embodied experiences and understandings which perpetuate that war, because the kinds of bodies the combatants now have demand violence, and apply this insight to other aspects of history and experience in other cultures, and other times?

Another fundamental issue of identity, gender and sexing, is perhaps the key area in the study of the thoughtful body. How bodies are identified and sexed, what criteria are used to determine the sexual status of bodies, and the way in which body parts are defined or ignored in the embodiment of gendered roles, are some of the issues which the study of embodiment needs to explore. Relationships between sexing and gendering practices, and other aspects of social life, such as the design of living space, the manner and rules governing talk, and the embodiment of ideals of gender form and meaning as expressed in men's and women's work, are some of the issues which a critical model of the body can begin to draw together into a unified field of study.

Finally, though not exhaustively, the question of what is, and is not, a body needs to be addressed. In this text I have been talking about bodies as I recognize them. That is, tangible and human in form. In the study of embodiment, it will be necessary to define the limits of the field of study and observation, by determining the embodied meaning of non-human bodies such as Samoan *aitu*, ancestors, and gods. When we talk about bodies, are there bodies we need to add to our scrutiny and consideration? These issues, like so many others, arise from what I see as a new path the study of embodiment can offer to anthropology. Such a study builds on anthropology's accomplishments as a discipline by taking it in new, and I feel, compelling directions.

The title of this chapter is poetic, a recollection of a line from a piece by William Blake. I chose it because, for me, the final aspect of the body which makes its study so challenging is that, not only is embodiment ongoing, it is instantaneous. In the moment we apprehend the presence of another body, we know everything we need to know about that body in order to see it. In an instant, we know its gender, its relative age, whether it is attractive or anomalous or a threat. The body before us is meaningful. In the time it takes light to fall on a body, to become visible, we have constituted it, and made it sensible, through our own embodied understanding of the world, and through the embodying efforts of the body before us, which make it observable, thoughtful, and suggestive.

Our ability to recognize and understand the bodies around us, and to present our own bodies in recognizable and comprehensible ways, are key moments when embodiment crystallizes our being in the world. In those moments, we engage the accumulated practice of being a body in what I feel is the most fundamental aspect of culture—experiencing, through our bodies, what the world means. But perhaps more important, we know, again through our body as a sensuous process and a thoughtful imagining, that that world must mean something. I have argued in this text for an anthropology of that moment of recognition and understanding, because grasping how that moment is possible can take us into the core of what being is, as a collaborative presence in the world.

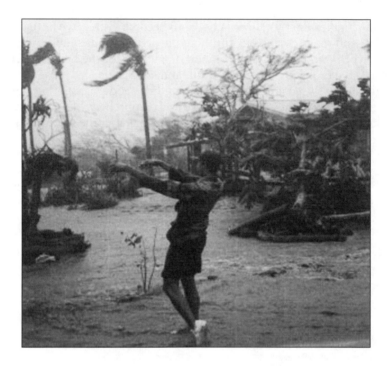

Coda

The picture is dark because the air, the wind, rain and light, are dark. It is a picture of a tall body, taken at the height of a cyclone. It is the middle of the day. He is standing, arms raise in front of him, standing on one foot. It looks like a dance, or a hex. I cannot tell exactly what he is doing. His body. The elements. They are both inventions, both compositions and Siaosi is standing there in that peculiar dance which is the apposition of the body and body the world moves in, punctuating that peculiar story about the invention of nature and the deconstruction of the real into the social and the social into the real. Siaosi is a body. The world is a body. Siaosi has a body and he also has the body of the world both in and on his body. That point, that pivot in this darkened photograph, that is the moment of presence and clarity we need to explore. Piece together. Take apart. Siaosi's body does not occupy space, it makes space in order to be a body. We need to untangle this making of space which is also the invention of the body moving through the space that bodies make, an invention which leaves us with this photograph of a tall Samoan boy, body posed in the heart of the body of the world he makes by being made. As I still only dimly understand, it is not the mats, it's the weaving.

Endnotes

Chapter 2 Endnotes

1. At the time of my original field work, the Independent State of Samoa, as it is now known, was officially known as the Independent State of Western Samoa, differentiating it from its companion islands, American Samoa, which remains a protectorate of the United States. Laying claim to the name Samoa has important political and nationalist ramifications for Samoans well beyond this current text.

2. I don't think it is possible to overstate the importance of AIDS in the intellectual history which informs the study of the body. HIV/AIDS so tragically inverts conventional expectations of the good and proper body, wherever the disease emerges, that its implications and complications for the study of culture will continue to be felt for decades. Herdt and Lindenbaum 1992 are the best early example of just how wide ranging and transformative AIDS has been, and continues to be, for the various intellectual and activist projects which shape the engagement between anthropology, anthropologists, and the world.

3. Boddy goes on to express a concern over "unintended essentialisms" in locating embodiment at the heart of cultural and social analysis, though it is unclear what risk essentialism poses to such an analytic strategy. Because the body is naturalized as a thing in itself, masking its productive and constructed character, it is fundamentally and unavoidably essentialized in lived practice. The task of an embodied approach to society and experience is not to simply be suspicious of essentialisms, but to problematize how they come to work as natural objects in specific cultural and historical milieu.

4. The literature on body image psychology, spanning more than 50 years of research, is summarized in Fisher [1986]. This area of study of the body has explored the idiosyncratic, cultural, and pathological, aspects of body experience almost exclusively in European or American contexts. I will not deal with psychological perceptions of the body here, however, because my main focus is on the larger relationship between embodiment, and cultural ideals and values. Psychological studies of Samoan body image, which I feel would contribute to the argument I will advance here, require specialized research methods. This is an area of the study of Samoan bodies I am pursuing in continuing research.

5. Some of the best work in this area have been gathered in Feher's three volume *Fragments for a History of the Human Body* [1989]. Of particular note, Knaufft's analysis of the poetics of body modification in Melanesia expands such studies from a focus on the aesthetics of design to a consideration of how these practices not only mark identity, but enact it as an ongoing process in societies where social identity is rapidly changing. Bynum discusses the relationships between food and gender in women's religious practices

in the late middle ages in Europe, linking the experience of the transubstantiated host of the Christian Eucharist to issues of women's power and social position in patriarchal societies [1989:160-219, and see also Bynum 1987]. Perhaps most important for future study of the body as a cultural and historical phenomenon, Duden provides a comprehensive annotated bibliography of body studies [1989:470-578].

6. For example, Fabrega [1993] explores how bio-psychiatry, because it is a practice of moral assessment of the qualities of the self, needs to be deconstructed as a knowledge practice in order to expose its body producing affect, while Comaroff [1993] argues that anatomists emphasis on the savage and simian qualities of Africans not only effected European perceptions of, and reactions to, African bodies, but also effected African's experiences of their own bodies.

7. The body aroused, or more compellingly, the body wanting to be aroused, that is the desiring body, has begun to engage researchers in tantalizing ways. Some of the most compelling work on embodiment comes out of attempts to "culturalize" and "historicize" the sexual body, in particular in that connection between bodies, identity, and the community of other bodies to which were are connect through the practices of constituting and enacting sexualities and sexual orientations. And so, for example, Holmberg [1998] argues for a non-canonical approach to the study of sexual desire, sexuality, and identity which frames the analysis in the everyday formation of popular culture as the lived space where myths of pleasure, sexuality, and power are enacted. McWhorter [1999] arguing from a deeply reflexive engagement with her own sexualized body, suggests that the predominance of developmental models of the bodies life, a form of which I apply uncritically here, are themselves forms of an objectifying gaze which fetishize the ongoing constructedness of the body and its self-relations, as part of system of surveillance and social control. And Parker et al. [1992] and Lancaster [1992] picking up and ideas emerging in European history and social analysis such as Mosse [1985], demonstrate how an embodied approach which focuses on issues of intimacy, sexuality and desire can contribute to a more comprehensive understanding of the way nationalism and national identity function as constraints on both embodiment and on historical process. These areas are ones which informs my current work on transient sexualities, and commodified identities among male street prostitutes in Canada.

8. I refer here to Berger and Luckman's [1967] work on the sociology of constituting the world; Gergen's [1985] review of the importance of the concept of social constructionism in psychology; Harre [1986] and Lutz [1988], whose work on the cultural constitution of emotional experience locates social constructionist studies in some of the most intimate aspects of a person's life; and Whitman's [1993] discussion of the practical value of social constructionist models in Western medical practice.

9. For example, Ochs [1988] on socialization, language acquisition, and cultural knowledge; Mageo's work on such issues as gender and sexuality [1992 and1998], spirit possession [1991], and the nature of self awareness in Samoa [1989 and 1998]; MacPherson and MacPherson's [1990] study of the history and current practice of "traditional" healing; and Duranti's [1994] examination of the constitution of political authority through speech acts.

Chapter 3 Endnotes

1. While the literature, and the debate, over colonial co-optation and subjection is vast, and recent debates over post-colonial history and historical consciousness is perhaps one of the most contentious fields in contemporary social theory and analysis, I will not insult my friends and colleagues in Samoa by dismissing their historical understanding as misguided and ignorant. Samoans have a sophisticated grasp of their history, of their place in global history, and of their participation in the histories to come. It would be disingenuous of me to not take seriously their experience and understanding of the transition to Christianity which is at the heart of contemporary Samoans sense of their national and global identities. However, I want to acknowledge that the question of colonial and post-colonial embodiment is a complex and contentious area of analysis, even if beyond the scope of this current book. Interested readers should see Helm [1998] for a fascinating discussion of the health of First Nations people in British Columbia, Canada, during the colonial and "post-colonial" periods, or Blunt and Rose [1994] for a discussion of social and moral geographies, embodiment, and the post-colonial.

2. This brief history of Samoan independence is based on my Samoan father's account. His own father was very active in the Mau, and Sei'a, my father in Samoa, was present during many of the meetings of the Mau, in the years leading up to independence.

3. The issue of what constitutes a corporate group in Samoa is complex, because the answer always depends on the circumstances. The most formal corporate group is the *'āiga potopoto*, but there are other corporate groups, including not only the smaller more intimate *'āiga*, but the household [similar to our nuclear family], the village, the political district and, occasionally, the nation as a whole. See Shore [1982] for a detailed discussion of the political and structural implications of different kinds of corporate groups in Samoa.

4. The complexity of the notion of claims to genealogical ownership of titles can only be hinted at here. Shore [1982] offers the most fulsome and detailed analysis, while Mageo [1998:110ff] offers a significant addition of analytic depth in here analysis of the Samoan discourses on power, authority, and stately persons. Because I do not intend to deal in great detail with gender in this current text, a key component of these genealogies involving relationships of descent along gendered lines—*tamafafine* [female] and *tamatane* [male] cannot be explored. However, it should be noted that embodiment, and in this instance, gendering and sexing, are insinuated in even the most abstract structures of Samoan social order, including the near mythical hierarchies of chiefs and their followers.

5. Shore [1982] provides the most detailed analysis of the *matai* system in Samoa, and I have relied on his account, combined with explanations of the importance of aspects of this system of leadership provided by my own informants.

6. I should note here that Mageo glosses *tautua* as rendering goods and services to a hierarchical superior, which in my interpretation over-emphasizes the relationships of status and rank in the *soa* connection. I say over-emphasizes, not because I think her reading is incorrect, but because it appears to fix too statically the ongoing calculations of rank and obligation in every day Samoan life. I would qualify her gloss by suggesting *tautua* is service to some hierarchical superior, whether real or potentially superior being a process of ongoing calculation. Indeed, the relationship of *tautua* can become inverted with person A standing in a *soa* relationship to person B under one set of circumstances, and then

having person B stand in a *soa* relationship to him or her under some other conditions. This suggests to me that the *soa* relationship is circular and reciprocal rather than hierarchical and expresses a mutuality of support rather than support in only a single direction.

7. Gell [1993] explores the tattooing complex throughout Polynesia, concluding that it was invariably associated with rank, or its acquisition, and was not, as Sparks [1965] and Marquardt [1984] argue, simply decoration or a way of attracting the opposite sex. The most detailed discussion of the process of tattooing in Samoa can be found in Forsyth [1983] and includes both a discussion of the relationship between tattoos and health, but also a thorough catalogue and analysis of tattoo designs. For a discussion of the relationship between tattoos and chiefly status in Samoa prior to European contact, see Franco [1991:128-134].

8. In a study of chiefly language, Duranti advances a parallel "moral flow" model of the embodiment of persons and space which confirms many of the conclusions I describe here [Duranti 1994]. His model argues that Samoan chiefly oration is one means Samoans have for mapping praise and blame as a way of deploying dignity in their everyday lives, an argument which coincides with my description here of the mapping of dignified village space.

9. Shore [1977] proposes that it is not unreasonable that *lēaga* is a combination of the negative marker *lē*, and *aga*, which can be roughly translated as socially good or appropriate.

10. There is a third form of Samoan, labelled by linguists as respect language, which is reserved for important public performances by *matai*. It is most often used at the openings of important meetings of *matai* or in formulaic presentations to the courts or to parliament. As such, its use is very rare.

Chapter 4 Endnotes

1. This is an ongoing project which examines, among other things, individual conceptions of organic body function. It grew out of long term research with persons at risk for HIV, in which I have been exploring how idiosyncratic biological models effect safe sex and other preventative practices among male street sex workers. While anthropologists have a longstanding tradition of mapping "local" theories of various cultural and practical matters, I want to stand back and ask a somewhat different question about how particular and idiosyncratic personal biological models give form and structure to any given persons health making, and to wonder how best to collect, analyse and situate these specific understandings in our understanding of health at a community level.

2. In contrast, Sahlins has suggested that the semen, and possibly the menstrual blood, of "royal" Hawai'ians may have been considered dangerous, and subject to taboos related to the enactment of political authority and rank in ancient Hawai'ian society [1985:3-26].

3. The incorporation of rice into the Samoan diet, which has accelerated throughout this century, is something many of the authors in Baker, Hanna and Baker noted was contributing to serious nutrition problems in both Samoan children and adults. As I discuss in the next chapter, boiled white food, such as taro, bananas and rice, is food of very high status both because of its colour, and because of its association with men who are usually the ones who prepare it. Many of my informants also "hinted" at a connection between these boiled white foods and semen, though their embarrassment made it difficult to pur-

sue this as thoroughly as I would have liked. What it suggests, however, is that during pregnancy and also during the first year or so of life, there is at an important symbolic continuation of the father's contribution of semen to the childs physical development through food choice.

4. Sexualized body images, as psychological phenomenon, are explored in Fisher [1989]. The question of standards and pathologies in body image experience across cultures is important because, as Kleinman [1980] reminds us, what is pathological in one culture may be normative in another. Exploration of a culturally sensitive approach to body image psychology, and its pathologies, is part of my own continuing research on gendered bodies in Samoa.

5. The passing of character traits such as temperament, intelligence and so on from parent to child is not the issue here. While Clement [1974], Gerber [1975] and Maxwell [1969] discuss this aspect of biology and self, it is unclear from my own research whether Samoans have a well developed model of the inheritance of non-physical traits. Rather, from my discussions, it was apparent that psychological traits are in fact derived from physical events such as eating the wrong foods, *aitu* attack, or injury during pregnancy. While my informants often talked about the character of some persons ancestor, for example commenting on how good or humble a person someone father may have been, and expressing surprise or disappointment that the son or daughter did not share these traits, this was not a reference to inheritance. Rather, the connection being expressed was contiguity. The son or daughter of a good and humble parent *should* have *learned* these qualities. That is to say, character traits are acquired rather than inherited. However, in interesting side issue in my own ongoing exploration of the making of good and proper Samoans is the extent to which the work on temperament and children's invention of the world around them initiated by Bruner [see, for example, Bruner and Haste 1987] can help understand differential outcomes in child socialization in Samoa, whatever the detail or complexity of Samoan models of temperament and inheritance.

6. Readers may be vexed by repeated references to this third sex. Even after nearly a decade of study, I remain vexed by it as well. In Chapter 5 I deal in somewhat more detail with this phenomenon, and so do not want to labour over it here. However, some things are striking. One is that this is a state recognized early on in a child's life, a reading of the body derived from the child's actual behaviour. Another is that the word, *fa'afafine* refers to a manner of being, rather than to a state or condition as do *tamatane* and *tamafafine*— a state of incompleteness. This may, however, be too fine a distinction. While Mageo [1998] seems most comfortable with the notion of *fa'afafine* as temporarily incomplete males, what I think these designations point to is process rather than specification. That is, all adolescents and young adults are in a state of motion between a near foetal, animal like condition, to dignified and obligated adulthood. Rather than reading incompleteness onto *fa'afafine* I think it is perhaps more fruitful to read process onto *tamatane* and *tamafafine*. To explore this further would require a different kind of the book than this one. However, readers interested in this issue should turn to Mageo's comprehensive analysis of gender and sexuality in Samoa [1998] or the Herdt's edited volume of studies of "third genders" in cross cultural perspective [1994].

Chapter 5 Endnotes

1. My informants would use the word *uma* in this regard. *Uma* signifies several things: completion, fruition, sufficiency. It is also used to correct children, so, for example, to silence a noisy child a care-giver might simply shout "*uma,*" simply meaning "enough." My experience of the word suggests its core meaning is something like "done, for now" but that is does not mean something is at an end. I do not think there is indeed a concept of "finished for all time," at least as it relates to social action, since in the ramifying model of action and consequence underlying *Fa'a Samoa*, a thing or event is both its own particular qualities and its consequences. This seems to me to be a Samoan version of the idea that the motion of a butterflies wings over the great wall of China is eventually related to a thunderstorm in the Sudan. Shore [1977] discusses the Samoan model of action most fully.

2. Several informants suggested the pattern of weight loss during childhood was a function of the slow emergence of one sexed substance as more important than the other in the bodies mechanical development. As I mentioned in the previous chapter, at around 12 either blood or semen comes to place a more central role in the bodies development. The process of redistribution of effect of body substances begins, for these informants, very early in childhood instead. Material I cannot deal with here but which offers interesting glimpses into the degree of pluralism which informs all ethno-biologies relates to the consequences when this redistribution fails. Indeed, as part of the emergence of a pathology model of homosexuality for some of my informants, they suggested that the trend toward *fa'afafine* retaining that sex well into full adulthood was a result of, as one minister put it to me, "too much blood and not enough semen in their bones." It should be noted here that, unlike many semen distribution complexes found elsewhere in the Pacific, for Samoans semen cannot be added to the body after birth. However, semen does have nutrient characteristics, though these appear, from the preliminary data I have gleaned from interview notes, to be restricted in their effect to adults and adults alone.

3. I want to thank Mike Evans for raising this issue, and sharing his understanding of the question of class in neighbouring Tonga, which has helped to shape my understanding of how, and why, this issue is becoming so important in Samoa.

4. This discussion of eating, sexing, and the meanings of food, is based on in depth interviews, and on detailed food intake data collected over a 28 day period in a sample of 18 households in six villages on Upolu.

5. A full and thorough discussion of food, eating, meals, and embodiment would require a separate book, so complex is this set of connected issues in Samoa, as it is elsewhere. The role of food in marking status, the meanings attached to different foodstuffs, the moral geography of growing, preparing, eating and sharing food are only some of the multiplying facets of this aspect of Samoan culture. And so I can only touch on these issues here, acknowledging the work of Wiessner and Scheifenhovel [1996] and Pollock [1992] as well as Mageo [1989b], and in particular discussions with Nancy Pollock, Heather Young-Leslie, Penelope Schoeffel and Dan Jorgensen in helping me begin to grasp this area of *Fa'a samoa*.

Chapter 6 Endnotes

1. See also, Shore [1982:241-242], where he discusses the orientations of particants in the *fono* in terms of the *tulafale* serving as the mouth for the head, represented by the *ali'i*. My point here is somewhat different, in that what I am describing, and will describe yet again in Chapter 8 when I discuss anatomy, is a proliferation of embodied models all built around the same core concepts of center and periphery, and all with the same relationship of increasing or decreasing dignity depending on where one is physically located in these socialized spaces.

2. For a detailed description of tattoo designs, and the implements and techniques of tattooing, see Handy [1971] and Marquardt [1984]. Gell [1993] offers a socio-structural and historical analysis of tattooing in Polynesia, though my own discussions of these practices are not consistent with his observations. A more detailed comparison between Gell's analysis and contemporary tattooing practices in Samoa is in preparation.

3. This apparently gendered difference in the expression or presentation of respect is striking because, from my experience, it is so unusual in Samoa. Further study of this aspect of gender and status in Samoa is needed.

4. Gilson [1970] and Goodman [1971] provide detailed discussions of the role of *aitu* in all aspects of Samoan life, including their religious significance in pre-European Samoa, and Handy [1927] is a comprehensive comparative review of religion in Polynesian societies, including the importance and function of spirit beings to these societies. While I am restricting my discussion here, and in the next chapter, to *aitu's* importance in punishment and illness, the significance of *aitu* in other aspects of *Fa'a Samoa* should be noted. *Aitu*, as either ancestors or their representatives, maintain a Samoan's kinship ties beyond death, and as such, have important implications for analysing what is and is not a body in Samoa.

Chapter 7 Endnotes

1. The *aualuma* and the *aumaga* are loose associations of untitled men and women who perform various kinds of work around the village, such as policing, the preparation of food for important ceremonial occasions, village building and clean up projects and so on. From my experience, these groups appear to come into existence as needed, rather than existing prior to some large or team oriented project arising. However, in some villages, these groups actually met as corporate groups to plan for, rather than simply respond to, the need for groups to perform large projects. Mageo [1998] suggests these groups once played important ceremonial roles.

2. But the a-social, and potentially anti-social space of the bush is also a space defined by social action, in this instance, by the social action which creates the boundaries between one kind of space and another. That act of making borders serves to make not only the space of the bush, but the spaces it is being differentiated from, ambiguous and open to contest and dispute. This ambiguity is built directly into the carefully demarcated system of socialized spaces in Samoa, part of the persistence of flux, if you will, which marks *Fa'a Samoa*.

3. Another word, *fa'auo*, was used by some informants to describe intimate conversations and activities. The word, which literally means the way or path of friends, embeds the importance of friendship dyads in Samoa, and links these to issues of privacy, as well.

4. There is a fundamental and controversial issue it is simply impossible for me to deal with here, related to the meaning, status, and practices surrounding viginity and gender in Samoa. Historical accounts, echoed by Mageo [1998 and elsewhere] suggest that marriage rites in Samoa once involved a ritual defloration of the bride as part of the compact between families. A practice of defloration, which approximates rape and involves young men crawling into young women's homes at night and violating their vagina in some way—referred to as sleep crawling or *moemoe* by some of my informants—is believed by many of my older informants to be a pressing social problem today, while most of my younger informants dismiss the idea as unthinkable. Female virginity is prized as an ideal, while for most of my informants male virginity is considered unimportant, even laughable. And yet, most of my informants also told me the virgin status of their wife at marriage was not a deciding factor, if a factor at all, for them. To further complicate matters, many of my older female informants told me they promoted virginity as a female virtue, but that they themselves did not consider it important, seeing it as a strategy deployed in securing good marriage matches. All this suggests to me that virginity is disconnected from such things as morality, propriety, and identity in ways which contrast sharply with the same ideals in North America, from which I draw my own experiences and values after all.

5. However, Coté [1994] does offer a detailed discussion of adolescence and adolescent sexuality, but his goal, which involves a critique of the controversial claims Derek Freeman has made against the work of Margaret Mead, is a hermeneutics rather than an erotics of Samoan sexual behaviour and identity. My analysis here attempts a different balance between these two objectives.

6. Many of my informants are angry with the way they feel they have been talked about by anthropologists, though few had actually read the work of Margaret Mead or others who have worked in, or dealt with, Samoa. This is a multi-leveled concern, and different actors have different agenda. For example, many university educated Samoans told me they felt Mead presented them as backwards simpletons, which they strongly contested. In everyday conversation, a concern which came up over and over was my informants feeling that Mead and others had presented Samoans are licentious and immoral, lazy and interested only in pleasure. This is an aspect of Samoans ongoing construction of *Fa'a Samoa* which needs further study and I am currently completing a paper on the question of Samoans talking about being talked about by others.

7. I will not explore, in detail, the content of Freeman's criticisms of Mead's work. Some of his arguments are about her methods, and these have already been successfully addressed by Holmes's restudy of Mead's informants in the 1950's and the 1980's [Holmes and Holmes 1992]. The main thrust of Freeman's argument with Mead, however, has been over the theoretical orientation of cultural relativism, a perspective with which Freeman disagrees. Readers are also directed to Cote [1994] and Orans [1996] for a discussion of this seemingly never ending debate. For my purposes here, the issue is not which of these two authors is right in their characterization of Samoan sexuality, because, I am arguing, they are both right. They are simply talking about two different things.

8. That *faleaitu* performances are often intensely sexual in their content bears this out and supports Mageo's suggestion that one of the things *faleaitu* accomplish is a release

from the stress of obligations and restrictions which surround aspects of everyday life in Samoa.

9. As I have noted throughout this text, conversations between men and women on issues which are private or embarrassing, are closely circumscribed in Samoa. I have indicated some of the limitations this imposes on my own data. What remains a fundamental mystery to me is Freeman's assertion that we treat the evidence of Mead's informants, a group of young women talking in private to another young woman, as duplicity, while we accept the absolute veracity of his data, reputedly drawn from conversations between older women, and a man. By his own admission, this kind of conversation contravenes fundamental rules of propriety and modesty in Samoa. I am convinced this aspect of Freeman's criticism of Mead is insupportable, not only on the evidence of Freeman's own description of modesty and cross sex relations, but from my experience dealing with these areas of privacy and embarrassment with my own informants. Discussing these sorts of issues with Samoans produces complex, and occasionally contradictory, evidence. It is scholarship of a most peculiar kind, which simply dismisses these contradictions as either lies or jokes.

10. As I noted in Chapter 3, the *soa* relationship is a core relationship through Samoan sociality, embodying support, authority and obligation, and the erotics of friendship and submission/control. I want to thank Reevan Dolgoy for reminding me of my tendency to over-simplify this complexity.

11. This parallels Davenport's [1965] observation that the absence of articulate repression of sex and sexuality in a society does not preclude regulation of these practices being strict, and even onerous.

12. The question of preferences, prohibitions, and the mechanics of sexual acts themselves needs to be explored as part of any attempt to understand sexing and gender. At the same time, in the time of HIV/AIDS, understanding the cultural logic of intimate acts of profoundly important. For example, the emergence of the HIV/AIDS epidemic in North America is substantially different in shape and scope because, at least among male urban homosexuals, certain high risk sex acts are preferred over other, lower risk activities than what one encounters in Britain. In Samoa, the strong dispreference for, though not necessarily disapproval of, anal sex and the pattern of acts in which *fa'afafine* are not as strictly enjoined to avoid this particular act will effect the pattern of epidemic emergence here and gives to the threat of HIV/AIDS a particular Samoan shape.

Chapter 8 Endnotes

1. Scarry [1985] offers a sometimes startling exploration of the idea of the body in pain unravelling the embodied, lived in world. I am extending her insight to the sick body in all its expressions.

2. However, an aspect of embodiment and culture as complex as health and healing can only be fully understood through collaboration. Along with my own field experience, four monographs on the professions of Samoan health and healing have also helped shape my understanding of these aspects of *Fa'a Samoa*. MacPherson and MacPherson [1990] not only provide a detailed description of contemporary Samoan healing techniques, their reconstruction of the history of healing in Samoa in the 20th century, has been instrumen-

tal in helping me to understand the nature of medical expertise in Samoa. In particular, their discussion of the flexibility of Samoan healers, and of their willingness to take advantage of "introduced" ideas and techniques, is a valuable corrective to the image of traditional healers are secretive and protective of their special status. Forsyth's [1983] discussion of healing and tattooing directly links diverse body practices into a single model of health and strength, while Kinloch's [1985] description of the importance of talking about illness, as an aspect of diagnosis and curing, has contributed to my understanding of how Samoans monitor health and disease through everyday conversation, highlighting the importance of illness-talk as a component of health culture. Finally, the papers gathered together in Baker, Hanna and Baker [1986] provide detailed bio-physiological data on Samoan health, and especially on issues related to the physical attributes of the good and proper Samoan body.

3. MacPherson and MacPherson [1990], provide a detailed and very comprehensive catalogue of ideas about anatomy held by Samoan healers, models which they note are generally shared by most Samoans. My own data, based primarily on interviews with patients, confirms this observation.

4. See also Butler [1993] and Alter [1992].

5. See, for example, Friedson [1970] and Stein [1990], for analyses of the sociology of medical expertise in the United States.

6. Perhaps the closest previous approaches to the body come to collapsing this fragmentation can be found in psycho-analysis, since it proposes that each person is persistently engaged in their own psycho-analytic surveillance and evaluation. The professional psycho-analytic encounter is thus only one kind of psycho-analytic field, one which taps into the overall flow of invention which psych-analysis seeks to clarify. See, for example, Freud [1989] and Anzieu [1989].

7. *Aitu* can also enter the body through the armpit and the mouth. They rarely enter women's bodies through the underarm, however, since the vagina is an easier passage. However, in some Samoans' understanding, *aitu* enter men's bodies through the armpit because the underarm area "mimics" the pubic region of women's bodies on the bodies of men. I heard this explanation often, but it was one of the more hotly disputed ideas about anatomy. Most people told me the underarm is a particular easy passage into the body, because the skin is weak in this region so that sweat can easily flow out of the body. Most people also agreed that the *aitu* rarely use the underarm to enter women's bodies.

8. One exception is weeping at funerals, by both men and women. This is considered reasonable since mourners are understood to be, at least temporarily, mentally deranged, and incapable of control.

9. It remains unclear if *musu* should be treated as a mental or physical derangement or condition. This stems in large part from the blurring of the distinction between physical ailments and conditions and psychological ones in Samoan health culture. However, Samoans do not presume to comment on the internal mental states of others, and in discussing emotional or cognitive disruptions, relate them as physical rather than psychic phenomenon. What can be known about a persons mental state is only what can be observed in the persons actions or in their physical condition since Samoans do not have a model of self which divides physical from psychic. That is, for Samoans there is no psyche as Western psychology understands it. Everything is body. One intriguing tributary issue in this regard is the way many of my informants conceptualized the Christian soul. For

them, the soul is the *manava*, the core of the body through which breath moves. This amorphous connection with the world through breathing is for them an organic connection which expresses in an embodied way their experience of being in the material world as transient, like a breath or a sigh.

10. There are some intriguing variations here as well. What is referred to clinically as dysthmia, a long standing form of clinical depression lasting longer than two years, which I encountered 4 times in Samoa, is not treated as a disease at all, but as a kind of moral and social bankruptcy. Post-partum depression, for which I have only sketchy comments and information, but which many older women told me was quite common, is not a mental disorder in their experience, but a normal reaction to the loss, during childbirth, of so much fluid body substance.

11. There is a special form of *aitu* attack, referred to as possession both by anthropologists and by my informants, which I have discussed, in relationship to punishment, in an earlier chapter. Possession is also implicated in illness, but I will not deal with that in detail here. Possession is a special form of spirit attack which might be conceived as resulting either from failure to attend properly to earlier less onerous attacks or illnesses, or from some extreme form of malefaction on the part of the patient or some member of her family. Most of the analytic discussion on spirit possession, for example Mageo [1998 and elsewhere] and Schoeffel [1979] focus on the important role gendering plays in the distribution and prosecution of spirit possession in Samoa, and see it as being a distinctive form of illness state. My own experience, at least in general, would confirm this. *Aitu* possession is most often associated with extreme conditions, including, as Mageo [1991] argues persuasively, conditions of general cultural transformation such as the period during WW II when Samoa was a base of operations for American and other troops fighting in the Pacific. Possession may be a mechanism for coming to accommodate extraordinary changes in Samoan culture by providing site at which the stress of transitions and transformations can be expressed and "treated." A different aspect of *aitu* possession may be related to what might be called the "christianization" of sexual behaviour in Samoa. As I noted in an earlier chapter, nocturnal emissions, or "wet dreams," were often spoken of as brief and uncontrollable possession-like encounters with *aitu* and many young men I have spoken with over the years have referred to the uncontrollably quality of their adolescent sexual urges as examples of a kind of possession as well, sort of a Samoan version of "the devil made me do it." At another level of remove from my discussion in this book, there appears to be a tenuous and not fully developed connection emerging between the trend toward *fa'afafine* adopting a life long, identity based sexual orientation and *aitu* possession among many of my informants. My ongoing research on the incorporation of *aitu* into Samoan sexual and moral rhetoric seeks to clarify these important practical and discursive changes.

Chapter 9 Endnote

1. Indeed, the Mau independence movement was formulated and led by *matai*. Factional divisions between groups of *matai* has been an aspect of Samoan politics all through its colonial and post-colonial history. Colonial administrators sought to undermine this factionalism by elevating some *matai* to positions of nation wide authority, but

so deeply entrenched are the family relations and the program of consensus which drives *matai* authority these efforts failed in their goal, though they succeeded in creating long standing rifts between alliances of *matai* which continue to foment contention in contemporary national politics in Samoa. Interestingly, the hegemony of *matai* authority, and the rhetoric and practice of that authority as an expression of consensus and humility, is so fundamental to Samoan social structure and social identity, the national level divisions between *matai* are more often than not expressed within a discourse of ethnicity, with the Chinese Samoans deployed as "cause" of these divisions by all sides in national debates. As I noted earlier, this parallels though does not necessarily mirror events in Fiji, where indigeneity and ethnicity are engaged as political strategies which mask the ultimate organs of power, the "traditional" chiefs. This cries out for further study.

References Cited

Abu-Lughod, Lila
1993   *Writing Women's Worlds: Bedouin Stories.* Berkeley: University of California Press.

Allardice, R.W.
1985   *A Simplified Dictionary of Modern Samoan.* Honolulu: Polynesian Press.

Alter, Joseph S.
1992   *The Wrestler's Body: Identity and Ideology in North India.* Berkeley: University of California Press.

Anzieu, Didier
1989   *The Skin Ego: A Psychoanalytic Approach to the Self.* New Haven: Yale University Press.

Baer, Hans, Merrill Singer and Ida Susser
1997   *Medical Anthropology and the World System: A Critical Perspective.* Westport: Bergen and Harvey.

Baker, Paul T., Joel M. Hanna and Thelma S. Baker [eds.]
1986   *The Changing Samoans: Behaviour and Health in Transition.* Oxford: Oxford University Press.

Baker, Paul T. and Douglas E. Crews
1986   *Mortality Patterns and Some Biological Predictors.* In Baker, Hanna and Baker, 1986, pp. 93-124.

Bakhtin, Mikhail
1984   *Rabelais and His World.* Bloomington: Indiana University Press.

Barnes, Wm. H. [ed.]
1889   *The Story of Laulii, A Daughter of Samoa.* San Francisco: Jos. Winterburn and Co.

Bateson, Mary Catherine and Richard Goldsby
1988   *Thinking AIDS: The Social Response to a Biological Threat.* Reading, MA: Addison Wesley.

Battaglia, Debbora
1990   *On the Bones of the Serpent: Person, Memory and Mortality in Sabarl Island Society.* Chicago: University of Chicago Press.

Becker, Anne E.
1995   *Body, Self and Society in Fiji*. Philadelphia: University of
         Pennsylvania Press.

Benedict, Ruth
1961   *Patterns of Culture*, with a new preface by Margaret Mead.
         Boston: Houghton Mifflin.

Berger, P.L. and T. Luckman
1967   *The Social Construction of Reality: A Treatise in the Sociology
         of Knowledge*. New York: Anchor.

Bindon, James R. and Shelley Zansky
1986   *Growth and Body Composition*. In Baker, Hanna and Baker,
         1986, pp. 222-253.

Blacking, John [ed.]
1977   *The Anthropology of The Body*. London: Academic Press.

Blunt, Allison and Gillian Rose
1994   Writing Women and Space: Colonial and Post-colonial
         Geographies. New York: The Guildford Press.

Boddy, Janice
1989   *Wombs and Alien Spirits: Women, Men and the Zar Cult in
         Northern Sudan*. Madison: University of Wisconsin Press.
1998   *Afterword: Embodying Ethnography*. In Lambek and Strathern
         [eds.], 1998, pp. 252-272.

Borofsky, Robert
1987   *Making History: Pukapukan and Anthropological Construc-
         tions of Knowledge*. Cambridge: Cambridge University Press.

Bourdieu, Pierre
1984   *Distinction*. Cambridge, MA: Harvard University Press.

Brewis, A.A., et al.
1998   Perceptions of Body Size in Pacific Islanders. *International
         Journal of Obesity Related Metabolic Disorders*, Feb 22(20):
         185-189.

Brody, Howard
1987   *Stories of Sickness*. New Haven: Yale University Press.

Bruner, Edward M.
1994   Essay: Abraham Lincoln as Authentic Reproduction: A Critique
         of Postmodernism. *American Anthropologist*, 96[2]: 397-415.

Bruner, J and Helen Haste
1987   *Making Sense: The Child's Construction of the World*. London
         and New York: Methuen.

Buck, P.H. [Te Rangi Hiroa]
1971   *Samoan Material Culture.* New York: Klaus Reprints [Bishop Musuem Bulletin #75].

Buckley, Thomas and Alma Gootlied [eds.]
1988   *Blood Magic: The Anthropology of Menstruation.* Berkeley: University of California Press.

Butler, Judith
1990   *Gender Trouble: Feminism and the Subversion of Identity.* New York: Routledge.
1993   *Bodies That Matter: On the Discursive Limits of "Sex."* New York: Routledge.

Bynum, Catherine Walker
1987   *Holy Feast and Holy Fast: The Religious Significance of Food to Medieval Women.* Berkeley: University of California Press.

Charlot, John
1990   Aspects of Samoan Literature II: Genealogies, Multi-generational Complexes and Texts on the Origins of the Universe. *Anthropo,* 86[1/3]: 127-147.

Clatterbaugh, Kenneth
1990   *Contemporary Perspectives on Masculinity: Men, Women, and Politics in Modern Society.* Boulder: Westview.

Clement, Dorothy Caye
1974   *Samoan Concepts of Mental Health and Treatment.* Ph.D. dissertation, University of California, Irvine.

Clifford, James
1988   *The Predicament of Culture: Twentieth-Century, Ethnography, Literature, Art.* Cambridge, MA: Harvard University Press.

Clifford, James and George E. Marcus
1986   *Writing Culture: The Poetics and Politics of Ethnography.* Berkeley: University of California Press

Comaroff, Jean
1985   *Body of Power, Spirit of Resistance: The Culture and History of a South African People.* Chicago: University of Chicago Press.
1993   *The Diseased Heart of Africa: Medicine, Colonialism and the Black Body.* In Lindenbaum and Lock [eds.], pp. 305-329.

Coté, James E
1994   *Adolescent Storm and Stress: An Evaluation of the Mead-Freeman Controversy.* Hillsdale, NJ: L. Erlbaum Associates.

Cox, Paul Alan and Sandra Anne Banack
1991   *Islands, Plants and Polynesians: An Introduction to Polynesian Ethnobotany.* Portland, OR: Dioscorides Press.

Crimp, Douglas [ed.]
1988   *AIDS: Cultural Analysis/Cultural Activism.* Cambridge, MA: MIT Press.

Csordas, Thomas J.
1990   Embodiment as a Paradigm for Anthropology. *Ethos,* 18: 5-47.
1993   Somatic Modes of Attention. *Cultural Anthropology,* 8: 135-156.
1994   *The Sacred Self: A Cultural Phenomenology of Charismatic Healing.* Berkeley: University of California Press.

Davenport, W.H.
1965   *Sexual Patterns and their Regulation in a Society in the Southwest Pacific.* In *Sex and Behaviour,* F.A. Beach [ed.], New York: John Wiley, pp. 164-207.

Davies-Floyd, Robbie E. and Carolyne Sargent [eds.]
1997   *Childbirth and Authoritative Knowledge: Cross-Cultural Perspectives* Berkeley: University of California Press.

de Certeau, Michel
1984   *The Practice of Everyday Life.* Berkeley: University of California Press.

Delaporte, Francois
1986   *Disease and Civilization: The Cholera in Paris, 1832.* Boston: MIT Press.

DelVecchio-Good, M., P.E.Brodwin, B.J.Good and A. Kleinman [eds.]
1992   *Pain As Human Experience: An Anthropological Perspective.* Berkeley: University of California Press.

Deutsch, Eliot
1993   *The Concept of the Body.* In Kasulis, Ames and Dissanayake, 1993, pp. 5-19.

Douglas, Mary
1970   *Natural Symbols.* Harmondsworth: Pelican.

Drozdow-St.Christian, Douglass
1994   *Coincidence and Likely Stories: Taking Note of Multiple Genders in Pacific AIDS Research.* Paper presented at the Annual Meeting, Association for Social Anthropology in Oceania, March 1994.
1993   *The Missionary's Problem: Misrecognitions of the Samoan Body 1 — The* Fa'afafine *and the Bodies of Men and Women.*

Paper presented to the Annual Meeting of the Association for Social Anthropology in Oceania, March 1993.

1992 *Framing the Flesh: Embodying Gender in Contemporary Samoa.* Paper presented to the 91st Annual Meeting of the American Anthropological Association, San Francisco, CA, Dec. 2-6, 1992.

Duden, Barbara
1989 *Repertory of the Body.* In Feher [ed.], 1989, vol. 3, pp. 470-578.
1991 *The Woman in the Body: A Doctor's Patients in Eighteenth-Century Germany.* Cambridge, MA: Harvard University Press.

Duranti, Alessandro
1992 Language and Bodies in Social Space: Samoan Ceremonial Greetings. *American Anthropologist,* 94: 675-691.
1994 *From Grammar to Politics: Linguistic Anthropology in a Western Samoan Village.* Berkeley: University of California Press.

Early, Evelyn A.
1993 *Baladi Women of Cairo: Playing with an Egg and a Stone.* Boulder: Lynne Rienner.

Epstein, Julia and Kristina Straub
1991 *Body Guards: The Cultural Politics of Gender Ambiguity.* New York: Routledge.

Fabrega, Horatio, Jr.
1989 *Biomedical Psychiatry as an Object for a Critical Medical Anthropology.* In Lindenbaum and Lock [eds.], 1989, pp. 166-187.

Farmer, Paul
1992 *AIDS and Accusation: Haiti and the Geography of Blame.* Berkeley: University of California Press.

Featherstone, Mike, Mike Hepworth and Bryan S. Turner [eds.]
1991 *The Body: Social Process and Culture Theory.* London: Sage.

Feher, Michel [ed.] with Ramona Naddaff and Nadia Tazi
1989 *Fragments for a History of the Human Body* [in 3 volumes]. New York: Zone.

Feierman, Steven and John M. Janzen [eds.]
1992 *The Social Basis of Health and Healing in Africa.* Berkeley: University of California Press.

Feldman, Allen
1991 *Formations of Violence: The Narrative of the Body and Political Terror in Northern Ireland.* Chicago: University of Chicago Press.

Ferguson, Harvie
1990   *The Science of Pleasure*. London: Routledge.

Finkler, Kaja
1991   *Physicians at Work, Patients in Pain: Biomedical Practice and Patient Response in Mexico*. Boulder: Westview.

Fisher, Seymour
1986   *Development and Structure of the Body Image* [Vols. 1 and 2]. Hillsdale, NJ: Lawrence Erlbaum Associates.
1989   *Sexual Images of the Self: The Psychology of Erotic Sensations and Illusions*. Hillsdale, NJ: L. Erlbaum Associates, 1989.

Fitzgerald, Maureen
1989   *Modernisation and the Menstrual Experience Among Samoans*. Ph.D. dissertation, University of Hawaii.

Forsyth, Claudia
1983   *Samoan Art of Healing: A Description and Classification of the Current Practice of "Taulasea" and "Fofo."* Ph.D. dissertation, United States International University.

Foucault, Michel
1972   *The Archaeology of Knowledge*. New York: Pantheon.
1973   *Birth of the Clinic*. London: Tavistock.
1979   *Discipline and Punish: The Birth of the Prison*. New York: Vintage.
1980   *History of Sexuality Vol. 1: Introduction*. New York: Vintage.

Fox, James W. and Kenneth B. Cumberland
1962   *Western Samoa: Land, Life and Agriculture in Tropical Polynesia*. Christchurch, New Zealand: Whitcombe and Tombs.

Franco, Robert W.
1991   *Samoan Perceptions of Work: Moving Up and Moving Around*. New York: AMS Press.

Frank, Arthur W.
1991   *For a Sociology of the Body: An Analytic Review*. In Featherstone, Hepworth and Turner, 1991, pp. 36-102.

Frankel, Stephen
1989   *The Huli Response to Illness*. Cambridge: Cambridge University Press.

Frankel, Stephen and Gilbert Lewis [eds.]
1989   *A Continuing Trial of Treatment: Medical Pluralism in Papua New Guinea*. Dordrecht: Kluwer Academic.

Freeman, Derek
1999   *The Fateful Hoaxing of Margaret Mead: A Historical Analysis of Her Samoan Research* Boulder: Westview.

1984   *Margaret Mead and Samoa: The Making and Unmaking of an Anthropological Myth*. New York: Penguin.

Freud, Sigmund
1989   *Five Lectures on Psychoanalysis* [translation, Strachey]. New York: Norton.
1993   *Sexuality and the Psychology of Love* [editor, Rieff]. New York: Collier.

Friedman, Richard C.
1988   *Male Homosexuality: A Contemporary Psychoanalytic Perspective*. New Haven: Yale University Press.

Fuss, Diana
1991   *Inside/out: Lesbian Theories, Gay Theories*. London: Routledge.

Gallagher, Catherine and Thomas Laquer [eds.]
1987   *The Making of the Modern Body: Sexuality and Society in the Nineteenth Century*. Berkeley: University of California Press.

Gallup, Jane
1988   *Thinking Through the Body*. New York: Columbia University Press.

Garber, Marjorie
1992   *Vested Interests: Cross-Dressing and Cultural Anxiety*. New York: Harper Collins.

Geertz, Clifford
1983   *Local Knowledge*. New York: Basic Books.

Gell, Alfred
1993   *Wrapping in Images: Tattooing in Polynesia*. Oxford: Clarendon Press.

Gerber, Eleanor Ruth
1975   *The Cultural Patterning of Emotions in Samoa*. Ph.D. dissertation, University of California, San Diego.

Gergen, K.J.
1985   The Social Constructionist Movement in Modern Psychology. *American Psychologist*, 40[3]: 266-275.

Gillison, Gillian
1993   *Between Culture and Fantasy: A New Guinea Highlands Mythology*. Chicago: University of Chicago Press.

Gilson, R.P.
1970   *Samoa 1830-1900: The Politics of a Multi-Cultural Community*. Melbourne: Oxford University Press.

Glassner, Barry
1988   *Bodies*. New York: Putnam.

Good, Byron J.
1994   *Medicine, Rationality, and Experience: An Anthropological Perspective*. Cambridge: Cambridge University Press.

Good, Carolyn G.
1980   *The Rat Brothers: A Study of the Brother-Sister Relationship in Samoa*. M.A. thesis, University of California at Berkeley.

Goodman, R.A.
1971   Some *aitu* Beliefs of Modern Samoans. *Journal of the Polynesian Society*, 80: 463-479.

Greenberg, David
1988   *The Construction of Homosexuality*. Chicago: University of Chicago Press.

Hallpike, Christopher
1986   *The Principles of Social Evolution*. Oxford: The Clarendon Press.

Hanna, Judith Lynne
1988   *Dance, Sex and Gender: Signs of Identity, Deviance and Desire*. Chicago: University of Chicago Press.

Handy, E.S.C.
1927   *Polynesian Religion*. Honolulu: Bernice P. Bishop Museum Bulletin #34.

Handy, E.S.C. and W.C. Handy
1971   *Samoan Housebuilding, Cooking and Tattooing [1924]*. New York: Krauss Reprints.

Hanson, Allan and Louise Hanson [eds.]
1990   *Art and Identity in Oceania*. Honolulu: University of Hawaii Press.

Harbison, Sarah F.
1986   *The Demography of Samoan Populations*. In Baker, Hanna, and Baker, 1986, pp. 63-92.

Harkin, Michael
1994   Contested Bodies: Affliction and Power in Heiltsuk Culture and History. *American Ethnologist*, 21[3]: 586-605.

Harre, R.
1986   *The Social Construction of Emotions*. New York: Basil Blackwell.

Helm, Mary-Ellen
1998   *Colonizing Bodies: Aboriginal Health and Healing in British Columbia, 1900-1950.* Vancouver: University of British Columbia Press.

Helman, Cecil
1991   *Body Myths.* London: Chatto and Windus.
1990   *Culture, Health and Illness* [Second Edition]. London: Wright.

Herdt, Gilbert and Shirley Lindenbaum [eds.]
1992   *The Time of AIDS: Social Analysis, Theory and Method.* Newbury Park: Sage.
1999   *Sambia Sexual Culture: Essays From the Field.* Chicago: University of Chicago Press.

Herdt, Gilbert [editor]
1982   *Rituals of Manhood: Male Initiation in Papua New Guinea.* Berkeley: University of California Press.
1984   *Ritualized Homosexuality in Melanesia.* Berkeley: University of California Press.
1994   *Third Sex, Third Gender: Beyond Sexual Dimorphism in Culture and History.* New York: Zone.
1999   *Sambia Sexual Culture: Essays From the Field.* Chicago: University of Chicago Press.

Hobsbawm, E.J. and T. Ranger [eds.]
1983   *The Invention of Tradition.* New York: Cambridge University Press.

Holmberg, Carl B.
1998   *Sexualities and Popular Culture.* Thousand Oaks: Sage.

Holmes, Lowell D.
1957   *The Restudy of Manu'an Culture: A Problem in Methodology.* Ph.D. dissertation, Northwestern University.
1958   *Ta'ū: Stability and Change in a Samoan Village.* Wellington, New Zealand: Polynesian Society.

Holmes, Lowell D. and Ellen Rhoads Holmes
1992   *Samoan Village Then and Now.* New York: Harcourt Brace Jovanovich College Publishers.

Hovdhaugen, Even
1987   *From the Land of Nafanua: Samoan Oral Texts in Transcription with Translation, Notes and Vocabulary.* Oslo: Norwegian University Press/ The Institute for Comparative Research in Human Culture.

Jackson, Michael
1983   Knowledge of the Body. *Man*, NS 18: 327-345.
1989   *Paths Toward a Clearing: Radical Empiricism and Ethno-
        graphic Enquiry.* Bloomington: University of Indianna Press.

Jameson, Fredric
1981   *The Political Unconscious: Narrative as a Socially Symbolic
        Act.* Ithaca, NY: Cornell University Press.

Jordan, Brigitte
1983   *Birth in Four Cultures.* Montreal: Eden.
1997   *Authoritative Knowledge and its Construction.* In Davies,
        Floyd and Sargent, pp. 55-79.

Jorgensen, D. [editor]
1983   Concepts of Conception: Procreation Ideologies in Papua New
        Guinea. Special Issue, *Mankind*, 14[1].

Kahn, Miriam
1986   *Always Hungry, Never Greedy: Food and the Expression of
        Gender in a Melanesian Society.* New York: Cambridge
        University Press

Kallen, Evelyn
1982   *The Western Samoan Kinship Bridge: A Study in Migration,
        Social Change and New Ethnicity.* Leiden: E.J. Brill.

Kasulis, T. with Roger T. Ames and Wimal Dissanayake
1993   *Self as Body in Asian Theory and Practice.* Albany: State
        University of New York Press.

Keene, D.T.P.
1978   *Houses Without Walls: Samoan Social Control.* Ph.D.
        dissertation, University of Hawaii.

Keesing, Roger
1984   Rethinking Mana. *Journal of Anthropological Research*,
        40[1]:137-156
1989   Creating the Past: Custom and Identity in the Contemporary
        Pacific. *The Contemporary Pacific*, Spring/Fall: 19-42.
1992   *Culture and Confrontation: The Kwaio Struggle for Cultural
        Autonomy.* Chicago: University of Chicago Press.

Kinloch, P.J.
1985   *Talking Health But Doing Sickness: Studies in Samoan Health.*
        Wellington: Victoria University Press.

Kirmayer, L.J.
1992   The Body's Insistence on Meaning: Metaphor as Presentation
        and Representation in Illness Experience. *Medical Anthropology
        Quarterly*, NS 6: 323-346.

Kleinman, Arthur
1980   *Patients and Healers in the Context of Culture*. Berkeley:
        University of California Press.

Kleinman, Arthur and Byron Good [eds.]
1985   *Culture and Depression: Studies in the Anthropology and
        Cross-Cultural Psychology of Affect and Disease*. Berkeley:
        University of California Press

Knaufft, Bruce
1989   *Bodily Images in Melanesia:Cultural Substances and Natural
        Metaphors*. In Feher, 1989, pp. 192-279.

Koskinen, Aarne
1968   *Kite: Polynesian Insights Into Knowledge*. Helsinki: Finnish
        Society for Missiology and Ecumenics.

Kramer, Augustin
1994   *The Samoan Islands Volume 1*. Honolulu: University of Hawaii
        Press.

Lacan, Jacques
1977   *Écrits: A Selection*. New York: Norton.

Lakoff, George and Mark Johnson
1999   *Philosophy in the Flesh: The Embodied Mind and Its Chal-
        lenge to Western Thought*. New York: Basic Books.

Lambek, Michael and Andrew Strathern [eds.]
1998   *Bodies and Persons: Comparative Perspectives from Africa and
        Melanesia*. Cambridge: Cambridge University Press.

Lancaster, Roger N
1992   *Life Is Hard: Machismo, Danger, and the Intimacy of Power in
        Nicaragua*. Berkeley: University of California Press.

Leder, Drew
1990   *The Absent Body*. Chicago: University of Chicago Press.

Lewis, Gilbert
1977   *Fear of Sorcery and the Problem of Death by Suggestion*. In
        Blacking, 1977, pp.111-144.
1980   *Day of Shining Red: An Essay on Understanding Ritual*.
        Cambridge: Cambridge University Press.

1993   *Some Studies of Social Causes of and Cultural Responses to Disease.* In Mascie-Taylor, pp. 73-124.

Lindenbaum, Shirley and Margaret Lock [editors]
1993   *Knowledge, Power and Practice: The Anthropology of Medicine and Everyday Life.* Berkeley: University of California Press.

Linnekin, Jocelyn and Lin Poyer [eds.]
1990   *Cultural Identity and Ethnicity in the Pacific.* Honolulu: University of Hawaii Press.

Love, Jacob Wainwright
1991   *Samoan Variations: Essays on the Nature of Traditional Oral Arts.* New York: Garland.

Lucile F. Newman [ed.] with the assistance of James M.
1985   *Women's Medicine: A Cross-cultural Study of Indigenous Fertility Regulation.* New Brunswick, NJ: Rutger's University Press.

Lutz, Catherine
1988   *Unnatural Emotions: Everyday Sentiments on a Micronesian Atoll and Their Challenge to Western Theory.* Chicago: University of Chicago Press.

MacCannell, J.F.
1986   *Figuring Lacan: Criticism and the Cultural Unconscious.* Lincoln, NB.

MacPherson, C. and La'avasa MacPherson
1990   *Samoan Medical Practices and Beliefs.* Auckland, New Zealand: Auckland University Press.

Mageo, Jeanette
1989   *Aga, Amio* and *Loto*: Perspectives on the Structure of Self in Samoa. *Oceania,* 59[39]: 181-199.
1989b   Ferocious is the Centipede: A Study of the Siginificance of Eating and Speaking in Samoa. *Ethos,* 17: 387-427.
1991   *Ma'i aitu*: The Cultural Logic of Possession in Samoa. *Ethos,* 19[3]: 352-383.
1992   Male Transvestitism and Cultural Change in Samoa. *American Ethnologist,* 19[3]: 443-459.
1998   *Theorizing Self in Samoa: Emotions, Genders, and Sexualities.* Ann Arbor: University of Michigan Press.

Marcus, George E. and Michael Fischer
1986   *Anthropology as Cultural Critique: An Experimental Moment in the Human Sciences.* Chicago: University of Chicago Press.

Marcus, Julie
1992   *A World of Difference: Islam and Gender Hierarchy in Turkey.*
        New Jersey: Zed Books.

Marquardt, P.
1984   *The Tattooing of Both Sexes in Samoa.* Papakura, New
        Zealand: R. McMillan.

Martin, Emily
1987   *The Woman in the Body: A Cultural Analysis of Reproduction.*
        Boston: Beacon.
1992   *Body Narrative, Body Boundaries.* In Grossberg, Nelson and
        Treichler, 1982, pp. 409-418.
1994   *Flexible Bodies: The Role of Immunity in American Culture
        from the Days of Polio to the Age of HIV/AIDS.* Boston:
        Beacon Press.

Mascia-Lees, Frances E. and Patricia Sharpe [eds.]
1992   *Tattoo, Torture, Mutilation and Adornment: The
        Denaturalization of the Body in Culture and in Text.* Albany,
        NY: State University of New York Press.

Mascie-Taylor, C.G.N. [ed.]
1993   *The Anthropology of Disease.* Oxford: Oxford University Press.

Maxwell, Robert John
1969   *Samoan Temperament.* Ph.D. dissertation, Cornell University.

McGrevy, N.L.
1973   *O Le Tatau: An Examination of Current Aspects of Samoan
        Tattooing to the Present.* M.A. thesis, University of Hawaii.

McLuhan, Marshall
1964   *Understanding Media: The Extensions of Man.* New York:
        McGraw Hill.

McLuhan, Marshall and Quentin Fiore
1967   *The Medium is the Massage.* New York: Bantam Books.

McWhorter, Ladelle
1999   *Bodies and Pleasures: Foucault and the Politics fo Sexual
        Normalization.* Bloomington: Indiana University Press.

Mead, Margaret
1961   *Coming of Age in Samoa: A Psychological Study of Primitive
        Youth for Western Civilisation.* New York: William Morrow
        and Co.
1969   *Social Organization of Manu'a* [Second Edition]. Honolulu:
        Bishop Museum Press Reprints.

Mechanic, David
1974   *The Comparative Study of Health Care Delivery Systems.*
        Madison: Health Economics Research Center, Center for
        Medical Sociology and Health Services Research, University of
        Wisconsin.
1978   *Medical Sociology* [2nd. Edition]. New York: Free Press.

Meigs, Anna S.
1983   *Food, Sex and Pollution: A New Guinea Religion.* New
        Brunswick, NJ: Rutgers University Press.

Milner, George
1966   *Samoan Dictionary.* London: Oxford University Press.

Morris, David B.
1991   *The Culture of Pain.* London: Jonathan Cape.

Mosse, George L.
1985   *Nationalism and Sexuality: Middle Class Morality and Sexual
        Norms in Modern Europe.* Madison: University of Wisconsin
        Press.

Moyle, Richard M. [ed.]
1974   Samoan Medical Incantations. *Journal of the Polynesian Soci-
        ety*, 83[2]:155-178.
1984   *The Samoan Journals of John Williams 1830 and 1832.* Can-
        berra: Australian National University.

Myers, Fred R.
1991   *Pintupi Country, Pintupi Self : Sentiment, Place and Politics
        Among Western Desert Aborigines.* Berkeley: University of
        California Press.

Naipaul, V.S.
1987   *The Enigma of Arrival: A Novel in Five Sections.* London:
        Viking.

Neitch, L and R. Neitch
1974   Some Modern Samoan Beliefs Concerning Pregnancy, Birth and
        Infancy. *Journal of the Polynesian Society*, 83[4]: 461-465.

Nichter, Mark [ed.]
1992   *Anthropological Approaches to the Study of Ethnomedicine.*
        Amsterdam: Gordon and Breach.

O'Hanlon, Michael
1989   *Reading the Skin: Adornment, Display and Society Among the
        Wahgi.* London: British Museum.

O'Neill, John
1985   *The Five Bodies*. Ithaca, NY: Cornell University Press.
1989   *The Communicative Body: Studies in Communicative Philoso-
        phy, Politics and Sociology*. Evanston: Northwestern University
        Press

Ochs, Elinor
1988   *Culture and Language Development: Language Acquisition
        and Language Socialization in a Samoan Village*. Cambridge:
        Cambridge University Press.

Orans, Martin
1996   *Not even wrong: Margaret Mead, Derek Freeman, and the
        Samoans*. Novato, CA: Chandler and Sharp.

Ortner, Sherry B. and H. Whitehead [eds.]
1981   *Sexual Meanings*. Cambridge: Cambridge University Press.

Parker, Andrew, Marry Russo, Doris Sommer and Patricia Yaeger [eds.]
1992   *Nationalism and Sexualities*. London: Routledge.

Parker, Richard G.
1991   *Bodies and Pleasures and Passions: Sexual Culture in
        Contemporary Brazil*. Boston: Beacon.

Parmentier, Richard J.
1987   *The Sacred Remains: Myth, History and Polity in Belau*.
        Chicago: University of Chicago Press.

Pawson, Ivan G.
1986   *Morphological Characteristics of Samoan Adults*. In Baker,
        Hanna and Baker, 1986, pp. 254-274.

Petrunik, Micheal and Clifford D. Shearing
1988   The "I," the "Me" and the "It": Moving Beyond the Meadian
        Conception of Self. *Canadian Journal of Sociology*, 13[4]: 435-
        448.

Pollock, Nancy J.
1992   *These Roots Remain: Food Habits in Islands of Central and
        Eastern Pacific Since Western Contact*. Laie, HI: Institute for
        Polynesian Studies.

Rosaldo, Michelle Z.
1980   *Knowledge and Passion: Ilongot Notions of Self and Social
        Life*. Cambridge: Cambridge University Press.

Rosaldo, Renato
1980   *Ilongot Headhunting 1883-1974: A Study in Society and
        History*. Stanford: Stanford University Press.
1986   *Culture and Truth: The Remaking of Social Analysis*. Boston:
        Beacon Press.

Roscoe, Will
1991   *The Zuni Man-Woman*. Albuquerqe: University of New Mexico Press.

Sahlins, Marshall
1985   *Islands of History*. Chicago: University of Chicago Press.

Sanders, Clinton R.
1989   *Customizing the Body: The Art and Culture of Tattooing*. Philadelphia: Temple University Press.

Scarry, Elaine
1985   *The Body in Pain*. New York: Oxford University Press.

Scheper-Hughes, Nancy and Margaret Lock
1987   The Mindful Body: A Prolegomenon to Future Work in Medical Anthropology. *Medical Anthropology Quarterly*, NS 1[1]: 6-41.

Schieffelin, Bambi B. and Elinor Ochs
1986   *Language Socialization Across Cultures*. Cambridge: Cambridge University Press

Schieffelin, Edward L.
1976   *The Sorrow of the Lonely and the Burning of the Dancers*. New York: St.Martin's Press.

Schoeffel, P.
1979   *Daughters of Sina*. Ph.D. dissertation, Australian National University.

Shore, Bradd
1977   *A Samoan Theory of Action: Social Control and Social Order in a Polynesian Paradox*. Ph.D. dissertation, University of Chicago.
1981   *Sexuality and Gender in Samoa: Conceptions and Missed Conceptions*. In Ortner and Whitehead, 1981, pp. 192-215.
1982   *Sala'ilua: A Samoan Mystery*. New York: Columbia University Press.
1989   *Mana and Tapu*. In *Developments in Polynesian Ethnology*, Howard, A and R. Borofsky [eds.], Honolulu: University of Hawaii Press, pp. 137-174.

Silverman, Kaja
1992   *Male Subjectivity at the Margins*. London: Routledge.

Sontag, Susan
1978   *Illness as Metaphor*. New York: Farrar, Strauss and Giroux
1989   *AIDS and Its Metaphors*. New York: Farrar, Straus and Giroux.

Sparks, R.W.
1965   *Polynesian Tattooing: The Techniques, Iconography, Patron-age, Profession and Esthetics.* M.A. thesis, University of Hawaii.

Stafford, Barbara Maria
1991   *Body Criticism: Imagining the Unseen in Enlightenment Art and Medicine.* Cambridge, MA: MIT Press.

Stair, John B.
1897   *Old Samoa or Flotsam and Jetsam in the Pacific Ocean.* Papakura, New Zealand: R. McMillan.

Stein, Howard F.
1990   *American Medicine as Culture.* Boulder: Westview.

Stigler, James W., Richard A. Schweder and Gilbert Herdt [eds.]
1990   *Cultural Psychology: Essays on Comparative Human Development.* Cambridge University Press: Cambridge.

Stoller, Paul
1994   Embodying Colonial Memories. *American Anthropologist,* 96[3-September]: 634-648.

Strathern, Andrew
1996   *Body Thoughts.* Ann Arbor: University of Michigan Press.

Strathern, Andrew and Pamela Stewart
1999   *Curing and Healing: Medical Anthropology in Global Perspective.* Durham, NC: Carolina Academic Press.

Strathern, Marilyn
1988   *The Gender of the Gift.* Berkeley: University of California Press.

Synnott, Anthony
1993   *The Body Social: Symbolism, Self and Society.* London: Routledge.

Taussig, Michael
1987   *Shamanism, Colonialism and the Wildman: A Study in Terror and Healing.* Chicago: University of Chicago Press.

Theweleit, Klaus
1987   *Male Fantasies Volume 1: Women, Floods, Bodies, History.* Minneapolis: University of Minnesota Press.
1989   *Male Fantasies Volume 2: Male Bodies: Psychoanalysing the White Terror.* Minneapolis: University of Minnesota Press.

Tiger, Lionel
1992   *The Pursuit of Pleasure.* London: Little, Brown and Co.

Turner, Bryan S.
1984   *The Body in Society.* Oxford: Basil Blackwell.

Turshen, Meredeth
1991 *Women and Health in Africa.* Trenton,NJ: Africa World Press.
1984 *The Political Ecology of Disease.* New Brunswick, NJ: Rutgers University Press.

Wagner, Roy
1975 *The Invention of Culture.* Englewood Cliffs, NJ: Prentice Hall.

Ward, R. Gerard and Paul Ashcroft
1998 *Samoa: Mapping the Diversity.* Suva/Apia: Institutes of Pacific Studies, University of the South Pacific and National University of Samoa.

Weiner, Annette B.
1992 *Inalienable Possessions: The Paradox of Keeping While Giving Away.* Berkeley: University of California Press.

Weiner, James
1988 *The Heart of the Pearl Shell: The Mythological Dimensions of Foi Sociality.* Berkeley: University of California Press.
1991 *The Empty Place: Poetry, Space and Being Among the Foi People of NewGuinea.* Bloomington: Indiana University Press.

Whitman, N.
1993 A Review of Constructivism: Understanding and Using a Relatively New Theory. *Family Medical,* 25[3]: 517-521.

Wiessner, Polly and Wulf Schiefenhovel [eds.]
1996 *Food and the Status Quest: An Interdisciplinary Perspective.* Providence, RI: Berghahn Books.

Williams, Walter L.
1986 *The Spirit and The Flesh: Sexual Diversity in American Indian Culture.* Boston: Beacon.

Winnicott, D.W.
1986 *Traditional Objects and Transitional Phenomena.* In *Essential Papers on Object Relations,* Buckley, P., New York: New York University Press, pp. 254-271.

Young, Katherine [ed.]
1993 *Bodylore.* Knoxville: University of Tennessee Press.

Zito, Angela and Tani E. Barlow [eds.]
1994 *Body, Subject and Power in China.* Chicago: University of Chicago Press.

Samoan Word Index

Index